Sex in the Outdoors

WHAT OTHERS ARE SAYING ABOUT <u>SEX IN THE OUTDOORS</u>

"If my library had to be reduced to one single book, there's no doubt in my mind it would be *Sex in the Outdoors*."

SMITH JONES,
CHAIRPERSON AND HEAD LIBRARIAN, INTERNATIONAL CONGRESS ON OUTDOOR SEX

"Until I found Buck Tilton's *Sex in the Outdoors*, I led a monkish life of woodland celibacy. Now, even on short dayhikes, I barely reach the trailhead before the fireworks begin. Thanks Buck!"

PIPPIN BRUCESTER
MANAGER, OMAHA BOOT REPAIR AND FERRET KENNEL

"While thru-hiking the Appalachian Trail several years ago, the closest I got to having sex was popping a blister on this hot chick's foot. After reading *Sex in the Outdoors*, though, I've hot-footed it with backcountry babes from Sweden, Italy, and West Virginia!"

LONG-TRAIL LOVER (FORMERLY KNOWN AS DRY CREEK HIKER)
ASSISTANT MANAGER, FEDERAL GOVERNMENT

"After reading *Sex in the Outdoors*, I've lost 20 pounds, am dating the man of my dreams, and I'm experiencing the best sex of my life, flat on my back on cold hard ground with little ice pellets hitting me in the eye while my toes turn blue."

JANET DULCIMER
SANDWICH ARTIST, NOME DELI

"For families and friends (and perhaps the odd stranger—maybe someone you've just met, maybe late at night, and maybe you don't even know their name) good clean fun is what this book is all about."

LESTER LESTOIL
PRESIDENTIAL CANDIDATE, EVERY FOUR YEARS

Sex in the Outdoors

second edition

by Buck Tilton, M.S.
with illustrations by Travis Bryant

MENASHA RIDGE PRESS

Library of Congress Cataloging-in-Publication Data

Tilton, Buck

Sex in the Outdoors/Buck Tilton. -2nd ed.

p.cm.

Includes bibliographical references and index.

ISBN 0-89732-579-6

1.   Sex instruction. 2. Outdoor recreation. 1. Title

HQ23.T56 2004

306.7-dc22   2004055159

Cover design by Travis Bryant

Text design by Travis Bryant and Annie Long

Illustrations by Travis Bryant

Menasha Ridge Press

2204 First Avenue South

Suite 102

Birmingham, AL 35233

Bed of Contents

Introduction to the Preface: A Disclaimer

"When ideas fail, words come in very handy."

—GOETHE

If anyone takes anything in this book seriously, they could wind up in serious trouble because (1) life is far too short to be taken seriously, and (2) if anything in this book bears any resemblance to anything factual, it's happened by serendipity. What follows is intended to be entertainment. If it happens to inspire any interesting ideas, that's great! But don't try this stuff in your own backyard, kids—at least, not without adult supervision.

Preface to the Introduction

"There are strange things done in the midnight sun . . ."

—ROBERT SERVICE

Anybody can have sex indoors . . . well, almost anybody. This book is not about the usual things sex books talk about, such as positions to do it in (although I guess it does mention some of those), routes to do it through (actually, perhaps, maybe, just a bit on those), or problems associated with doing it at all (except briefly in passing). These issues are just about the same no matter where you go . . . or come. This book is a light-hearted look at sex in the outdoors.

To be more accurate, this book was about sex in the outdoors—at least the first version was. This book, the new version, is about new and improved sex in the outdoors. A lot of recently discovered or deduced information is included, almost all of it entirely irrelevant, but, as with the first version of this book, that didn't stop me. If you read the first version, thanks a lot, and if you're thinking about buying this version, please do. I really need the money.

Buck Tilton

Introduction

"Truth is erotic."

—Margo Anand

Why write a book about sex in the outdoors? To tell the truth, when I confided to a few select friends and colleagues that I was working on this book (I was seeking interesting anecdotes, not bragging . . . at least that's what I told them), the most common response was: What in hell for? So I came up with this answer: If you're one of those people who's content to flounder along as you always have, possibly putting yourself and maybe other people in a risky situation, ignorant of your impact on a fragile ecosystem, oblivious to the possible variations that would make life much more interesting, unaware of the subtle context in which you are doing "it," and out of touch with higher philosophical thought that gives meaning to otherwise merely sensual behavior, then this book is not for you. But, if you are among the enlightened minority who prefer to enter the outdoor world prepared to protect yourself, sensitive to not leaving even footprints (let alone butt-prints), desirous of enjoying a full variety of experiences, and being in harmony with natural surroundings while your consciousness is raised to new heights, then this book is for you. This book may also be for you if you bought a bottle of wine but your date canceled out for this evening, there's nothing good on TV, and you're looking for something amusing to read.

Why write a book about sex in the outdoors? The notice on my kitchen wall reminds me daily that "Good lovin' don't last, good cookin' do!" But that isn't necessarily so. The point is this: There's a difference between a delicately seasoned and carefully prepared filet mignon and a hunk of beef blackened over a dung fire. Good cooking, like good sex, requires preparation. It's difficult to make a hollandaise sauce by trial and error. Although, admittedly, it might be more fun to cook up some outdoor sex through experimentation, there is a backpack-full of reasons to have a guidebook. The main reason is this: Who wants to eat a burned hunk of dung-smoked beef?

Why write a book about sex in the outdoors? For some the question might arise from simple unfamiliarity with the wild. Most people have, at least, a passing knowledge of sex, but they go into the great outdoors only occasionally—or not at all—and have thought little of putting the two together. (*Note:* This is especially true of people whose outdoor experiences are limited to Scout outings and family excursions in a huge walled tent.) For some the days of an outdoor trip are filled with making and breaking camp, moving from one place to another, preparing and eating meals, dealing with the weather, and, generally, squeezing as much non-sexual activity into the hours as possible. However, with a little planning, the sly smile of fickle fate, and some determination, anyone can squeeze some sex into every outdoor adventure. You don't have to leave home without it.

Why write a book about sex in the outdoors? Somebody had to do it—and I didn't have anything, or anyone, to do this weekend.

Sex in the Outdoors

A Brief History of
Sex in the Outdoors

*"Those who are ignorant of history are doomed to make the same
stupid mistakes again."*

—MY MOTHER, SHORTLY AFTER MY FIRST BIRTHDAY

Somewhere between four and five bazillion years ago, give or take a wild weekend or two, our hirsute ancestors got a little chilly. As the glaciers descended from the poles, "shrinkage" and "shooting bullets" entered the lexicon. Driven from a lush life well off the ground in the leafy trees that had always been home, they began to move south, where it was warmer, onto the vast grassy savannas of what is now known as Africa. Shuffling along on hands and feet proved painfully slow, but all the other creatures of the savanna were doing it, and anyway, pre-human brains were fairly small and not especially creative. Eventually, however, somebody starting walking upright, it caught on, and humans became bipeds. Becoming bipedal was, perhaps, the most critical moment in the development of sex-as-fun, as opposed to the old concept of sex-as-merely-reproduction-of-the-species.

Prior to bipedalism, people's physical views of each other were limited: a hunched over clump of matted hair and maybe a hairy-butt shot now and then. Sex was an instinctual urge, kind of like the poodle humping the cat—over in moments and less satisfying than the discovery of a banana or a mango. At this time the only warm fuzzy feelings occurred during the sex act itself. But, suddenly, everyone's sexual organs were hanging out or otherwise on display for all the world to see. Individualism began to take on a wholly unique meaning. This new view began to tingle a few primitive imaginations. Added to the visual impact of being bipedal was the fact that arms and hands, previously used most of the time for clinging to tree limbs, now had hours and hours of spare time. And there wasn't an awful lot to cling to on the African savannas. Furthermore, remember, it was still chilly, particularly at night, and temperature had a definite and substantial effect on the history of sex in the outdoors (see Chapter 7: Environmental Exposure). One frosty night, long after the mating season had ended, a pre-human, probably a male (since males had less body fat and cooled off quicker), suggested to another pre-human, probably a female (since the visible body parts were different and more interesting), that they have sex, just for fun. She went for the idea, the whole idea caught on, and, bless their long-departed souls, it continues today. *Primitive Opening Line:* "You want bite my banana?"

Little is known about sex in the outdoors over the next few million years. One of the few truly relevant discoveries, which got almost no publicity, is credited to the British paleontologists Louis and Mary Leakey, who, in 1959, recovered some of the oldest remains of primitive humans. This particular discovery, from the Olduvai Gorge in Tanzania, East Africa, dates from approximately 14 million years ago. It is apparently a grave of a socially high-ranking *Ramapithecus,* containing the complete mummified leftovers of a male, short of stature but impressively long on body parts associated with sex.

"Ram," it seems, was buried with several females, all with curious smiles frozen on their desiccated faces. Bone analysis confirmed that Ram died of exhaustion. Cause of death in the females has, at this writing, not been established. Although the evidence is slim, it certainly appears as if science may be way wrong about its long-held modern belief that desire to please a mate sexually is a recent evolutionary phenomenon (ignoring the feminist movement, of course). This one discovery added new and substantial weight in support of those who question the sincerity of oft-proffered assurances by females that "size doesn't matter."

Since humans have apparently reproduced throughout history and since "indoors" is a somewhat recent concept, many "sexperts" conclude that humans have a rich history of sex in the outdoors. But let's look at the facts. Archeologists have unearthed many artistic, and frankly pornographic, reproductions of human sexual activity. These discoveries, however, virtually all come from past metropolitan centers of civilization, i.e., cities, with the exception of a few crude, inconclusive cave-drawings here and there. Very little evidence inidcates that there has been a "rich history" of sex in the outdoors. It is much more believable that the sex acts pictured in those ancient reproductions (see *National Geographic Magazine*) were practiced only in pockets of human groups as an aberration of normal behavior, and those pockets of humanity, given what is evident today, quickly developed cities. Perhaps sex in the outdoors back then was just too dangerous to be a common, everyday occurrence. Perhaps the danger of exposure to a bitterly cold environment or the danger of exposing one's position to a potential enemy or carnivore were too great for a lot of sex to take place outdoors. After all, those same dangers exist today. And the lack of a lot of outdoor sex could explain why it took so long for the population to explode. The best hypothesis that can be scientifically stated is this: Nobody knows for sure. But life is full of uncertainties, and these uncertainties have made research for this book a whole lot more interesting.

To bring the history of sex in the outdoors a bit closer to home, let's take a look at eastern Massachusetts, shortly after the arrival of the Pilgrims. Before escaping from the religious intolerance of England, and what with it being the era preceding the Industrial Revolution, the Pilgrims, at least the wayward ones, most assuredly had some experience with rural sex (there were, after all, baby Pilgrims), but not with true sex in the outdoors as it is understood today. The first written record of any European's involvement in true sex in the outdoors comes from the splinter group, called Puritans, who moved up the coast to Salem some years after the landing at Plymouth Rock. (*Note:* Pre-Puritan sexual innuendoes, such as Leif Ericson's blond-haired –blue-eyed influence on Canadian Eskimos, and Columbus' contribution to the transatlantic distribution of certain viruses and bacteria, come to the pages of history through oral history and not the written word.) From Salem, the wilderness, the true outdoors, was close at hand . . . approximately 100 yards away. Occasionally, couples would accidentally find themselves outdoors, usually on a Saturday, the day allotted for reproduction of the species. Since it was Saturday, and the Puritans were creatures of habit, these few attempted to reproduce the species and, in so doing, made a fascinating discovery, namely that sex in the outdoors, unlike the quiet, cloistered sex of town, could be fun. The town fathers, being well-versed in intolerance, adept at voyeurism, and more than a little jealous, recognized the giggling as a real and present threat to their well-ordered society. So, in order to not over-educate the people, the term "witchcraft" was conjured up as a euphemism for sex in the outdoors. The subsequent fatal dunkings and burnings-at-the-stake effectively eliminated a budding sex-in-the-outdoors intelligentsia and negatively influenced public opinion concerning sex for years and years to come. In fact, that influence is still felt today. It was not until centuries later, after Kevin Costner filmed *Dances With Wolves,* that folks once again learned what most Native Americans always knew about the joys of sex in the outdoors.

Definition from the 1898 *Universal Dictionary of the English Language:*

Sex. s. [Fr. *sexe,* from Latin sexum, accus. of *sexus* = sex, prob. lit. = a division, from *seco* = to cut. Spanish & Portuguese *sexo,* Italian *sesso.*]

A. ORDINARY LANGUAGE

1. The distinction between male and female; the physical difference between male and female; that property or character by which an animal is male or female. Sexual distinctions are derived from the presence and development of the characteristic generative organs of the male and female respectively.

2. Womankind, by way of emphasis, and generally preceded by the term "the other."

3. One of the two divisions of animals founded on the distinction between male and female.

B. BOTANICAL LANGUAGE

A distinctive peculiarity of some flower or flowers, as bearing a stamen or stamens, and therefore being analogous to the male sex in animals, or bearing a pistil or pistils, and thus being analogous to the female sex.

As one can see by this 100-year-plus-old definition, sex has always *been . . .* but just what exactly it *was,* was not very clearly defined. With the plants, writers courageously used terms bordering on turn-of-the-century botanical pornography, terms such as "pistil" and "stamen," but with animals, i.e., humans, they wimped out with "characteristic generative organs" to describe sex. "Sex" was apparently not a word describing a performance, something that someone actually *did*, until later in the twentieth century, although most everybody assuredly had an interest in fooling around. If this book had been written by Charles Dickens, it would probably have been entitled *How to Have Characteristic Generative Organ Contact in the Outdoors.* Undoubtedly, it, too, would have been a bestseller.

In 1983, well into the modern era of thought and expression, a group of outdoor-oriented physicians in California founded the Wilderness Medical Society (WMS). WMS is dedicated to ". . . serving the medical interests of the outdoor and wilderness community," and now has thousands of members. Unfortunately, both Masters and Johnson live in the Midwest, were not among the founding fathers or mothers of WMS, and have had no noticeable influence on the Society. Despite the obvious need for one, the Wilderness Medical Society has no standing committee on sex in the wilderness. Its research-based *Journal of Wilderness Medicine* offers a quarterly dose of mind-expanding articles such as: "Monoclonal antibody detection of *Giardia lamblia* cysts in human stool by direct immunofluorescence." If the outdoor experts want to dip their hands into relevant research, how about a little sex in the outdoors, instead of shit?

So, as one can see, the history of sex in the outdoors lies shadowed by passive avoidance and active squelching of useful information. There does exist, however, a voluptuous body of knowledge gleaned from first-, second-, and third-hand reports that shed some light on this most fascinating subject. Much of this knowledge is contained within the pages of the book you hold in your hands. May it throw some candlelight into the seductive shadows.

Why Have Sex in the Outdoors?

"Do bears poop in the woods? You bet. But that's not all they do!"
—SMOKEY THE BEAR

More and more people are striving toward a closer relationship with the wild and good earth that birthed all life (and, just as a reminder, the prelude to all life is sex). Henry David Thoreau and John Muir wannabes across this great land understand on a gut level, that humanity has moved too far from its wilderness roots. Green individuals by the millions are actively seeking to reverse this trend by spending spare moments, weekends, and extended periods of time in the outdoors. This process of reconnecting to the natural world entails becoming familiar with one's natural activities in a wilderness setting, so that the things one does naturally indoors become things one does naturally outdoors. At its best, sex in the outdoors should be exceptionally normal. At its very best, sex in the outdoors should be normally exceptional. The point is this: Since sex is normal, sex in the outdoors should be normal. It's time to get sex out from underneath the covers and back in the open where it belongs.

An Expression of Oneness with Nature

Sex is a many-splendored thing. One of the splendored things sex in the outdoors can be is an expression of oneness with nature, perhaps the most beautiful expression. Like most species, humans have evolved naturally into a physical shape that lends itself to sex. Almost every other species on this earth does "the wild thing" in the natural world—outdoors—and some of them are doing it somewhere right now, even as you sit reading this compendium of silly words about it. If you really want to re-establish your active membership in the brotherhood and sisterhood of all fauna (and flora, for that matter), you *should* be having sex in the outdoors. Next time you're doing "it" in the outdoors, think of your act as a ceremonial rite, a bonding of yourself to the natural world. Let yourself be in contact with the rhythm of the universe through the rhythmic movement of your personal dance of this most natural act. Let yourself feel, through your emotional high, the threads connecting you to the cosmos. Let yourself join, through your coming together, the fertile continuum of all life—even if you've decided to put a stopper in, or on, your own personal fertility.

An Expression of Oneness with Another Oneness

Since it is impossible for any two people to draw physically closer together than when they have sex, it has been argued that there is no greater expression of oneness between a twoness than sex. If you're already into feeling universal rhythms and cosmic threads because you're outdoors, then this expression of oneness with another oneness should, understandably, reach new heights. Of course, it can also be argued that sex in the indoors can be just as expressive . . . but the view isn't as good.

An Expression of Ecosensitivity

For those individuals with a growing sense of concern about humanity as a destructive force among fragile ecosystems, and for those whose concern has led to an inclination toward the preservation of dwindling wild lands, it may be helpful to realize that sex in the outdoors can be a most expressive way of demonstrating ecosensitivity. In fact, sex in the outdoors may be the most environmentally sound activity in which one can engage while in pristine wilderness areas. Strip poker, for example, is far less disruptive than strip mining. (*Note:* There is that one notable exception from Montana in the early 1960s where an entire tract of virgin forest bordering a hippie commune was decimated in a single night.) Despite claims from the ecofringe crowd, there is absolutely no evidence that sex in the outdoors contributes to acid rain in any manner whatsoever. Neither does it have a detrimental effect on the ozone (with the exception, once again, of that one night in Montana). No other species has ever been pushed to extinction by human sex in the outdoors, nor has another species even been endangered—although a few have admittedly been embarrassed. (*Note:* More information about embarrassed species may be obtained from the U.S. Department of Agriculture. Ask for the Embarrassed Species List.) If one chooses location and technique carefully, and observes a few basic rules of etiquette, long-term alteration of watersheds and weather patterns can be avoided, and the creation and distribution of toxic wastes can be eliminated (see Chapter 9: Outdoor Sex Etiquette). Remember: Only you can prevent forest fires!

A New Dimension

For many city folk, there's something mysterious and fascinating about the sort of people who go wandering into the wild places. Those of you who are among the wanderers-in-wild-places, and who could also use an additional dimension to your dull and in-desperate-need-of-an-improved-image sex life, consider this: There are possibly millions of would-be partners in the cities, fascinated by the mystique surrounding *you* (even though you know better), who just might be snookered into a foray into the wild. This very same person, who rolls his or her eyes behind your back when you make those tired, predictable, citified come-ons in the office, may thrill to the suggestion of a moonlight hike up Pike's Peak. Somehow, it triggers a different response than your offer of a midnight stroll through Central Park . . . unarmed. *Opening Line to Remember:* "How 'bout we go down on, er, I mean, to the wildlife preserve this weekend, Doris?"

The corollary to the above idea is this: Sex in the outdoors can also bring an added dimension to your otherwise wild but increasingly-difficult-to-maintain-the-image-of-sex life. For those who expend lots of energy creating and maintaining a grandiose public image of their sex life, there's always the danger of running out of material. You can only relate so many variations on your urban/suburban sexual experiences to fellow travelers on the subway before the crowd starts to yawn. Outdoor sexual scenarios, on the other hand, are virtually limitless, and offer, additionally, the aura of the exotic and primitive (see Chapter 12: Testimonials: We Did It Our Way). Even a mediocre storyteller can get great mileage out of the wilderness milieu. After all, how many people actually know how far it is up Pike's Peak?

As Therapy

The great vices of today seem to be (1) struggling to be on time, (2) struggling to make the best use of time, and (3) struggling in a brief span of time to "achieve" and "succeed." What all this struggling produces is unhappiness, lack of peace, disassociation, and, finally, in the extreme, a bundle of psychotic disorders. But what a dynamic combo sex and the outdoors can be to reduce stress and improve one's self image! Ah, the healing power of the natural world combined with the healing power of the sex act. You may find here the ultimate therapeutic effect. Of course, many people have found this tack never works, but, hey, it's worth a try. *Opening Line to Remember:* "Let's go out to the national park, Sweetie, and we can both reduce a little stress!"

Warning! Outdoor Sex Addiction

There is a force that draws thousands of people to the dark side of sex in the outdoors. Many people walk that thin line that separates fun and fanaticism. Sex in the outdoors can be habit forming. In fact, sex in the outdoors can be addicting. If you become hooked, outdoor sex can unravel the social fabric into which your days are woven, disrupting your whole life. Moderation, as in all things, is strongly advised. Signs of sex-in-the-outdoors addiction include but are not limited to:

1. Having constant thoughts of sex in the outdoors (for example, where should I go next, and should I bring a tent or a tarp?), to the point that the thoughts interfere with your work and your relationships.

2. Having to have sex in the outdoors regularly to maintain a personal sense of well being.

3. Being overwhelmed by physiological and psychological depression if you don't have sex in the outdoors regularly (a.k.a., withdrawal).

4. Having to have sex in the outdoors more and more often in progressively larger doses to achieve the desired effects.

5. Having sex in the outdoors to excess, so you're exhausted, hung over, and generally wasted on Monday morning.

6. Leaving your Denver office early so you can have sex in Wyoming's Encampment River Wilderness on your way home to Colorado Springs.

7. Growing trees in your bedroom.

If you know someone, or know someone who knows someone, who might be addicted to sex in the outdoors, the following recommendations are strongly . . . well, recommended:

1. Explain in a calm, quiet manner to the person suffering sex-in-the-outdoors overdose or withdrawal that you are there to help. Remember, even though this person may be acting irrationally or inappropriately, she or he is almost always very frightened.

2. Maintain eye contact with the person, but do not look at any other body parts.

3. Wear protective gloves, goggles, mask, gown, and boots, if there is any chance of contacting this person's bodily fluids.

4. Protect yourself from an attack by this person (with a cast-iron chastity belt, working as often as not).

5. Gather as much information as possible (for example, when the person last had sex in the outdoors, how often he or she has sex in the outdoors, the routes of administration, and the most often-used geographic areas), in case you have to refer this person to professional help.

OSAA

Outdoor Sex Addicts Anonymous (OSAA) chapters are opening up all across the United States (and in a few other countries). For the address and phone number of the chapter nearest you, contact: OSAA National Office, 1849 C Street NW, Washington, D.C. 20240 (www.outdoorsex addictsanonymous.org).

Getting in Shape for Sex in the Outdoors

"Whatever else can be said about sex, it cannot be called a dignified performance."

—Helen Lawrenson

If you're under the age of 30, you can skip this chapter because you're most likely in good enough shape already. What nature provided you with still works all night long—and most of the day. If you're male, however, and you've noticed that watching a pair of tight, really brief hiking shorts walk past doesn't tighten *your* hiking shorts as much it used to, read on. If you're female, it is not known, at this writing, what to notice you don't notice as much of—but you can keep reading, too.

Physical Fitness for Fooling Around

Many people put hours and hours into choosing and packing the right gear and food, while forgetting that the basic piece of equipment for sex in the outdoors is made of flesh and blood. As with any other outdoor adventure, your body needs to be honed for sex. Lack of physical preparation may lead to premature exhaustion (pooping out before the fun really begins). Signs of poor fitness include but are not limited to: (1) saying you want to enjoy the rest break on the trail longer because the view is good, when the truth is you can't stand up, (2) saying you have a desire to watch the sunset, when the truth is you don't have the energy to crawl into the tent, and (3) getting breathless while undressing when you're alone. As a guideline, the American Council on Outdoor Sexual Fitness says that if you feel the need to lie down and rest after shrugging into your pack at the trailhead, you're probably in less than adequate physical condition for fooling around. Sex, in other words, is a matter of muscle and sweat, and the more of both the better.

As a bonus, it has been proven by scientific types that exercise gives a boost to the feel-good chemicals that your body manufactures. This has been spoken of in such terms as the runner's "high." Weight lifters sometimes speak of the same feeling as a "clean and jerk," but the devoted sex enthusiast, male or female, will know it by the term "erection." Many people indeed report feeling horny after a period of exercise, especially if they have been exercising in the nude, and very especially if they have been exercising in the nude with a partner who is also nude. *Opening Line to Consider:* "Spot me on this one, will you, Honey?"

ENDURANCE TRAINING

Any of the cardiovascular exercises—walking, jogging, swimming, biking, skiing—will work for overall conditioning for sex in the outdoors. These types of exercises will allow you to keep going longer. Holding your breath while doing these exercises will really help you prepare for prolonged sexual experiences. Doing these types of exercises naked will prepare you in other ways, such as helping you focus on the reason why you're doing all this exercising anyway. It should go without saying, but here it is anyway: The very best exercise to prepare you for extended periods of sex is extended periods of sex. As Sophocles said almost 3,000 years ago: "You may think you know a thing, but you have no certainty until you try."

STRENGTH TRAINING

A few push-ups and sit-ups, several of each several times a week, will help keep you in shape for general strength requirements during outdoor sex, such as rolling over and shaking your partner until he or she wakes up. Some people find muscle-specific strength-training exercises valuable, such as

 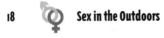

squeezing a basketball between your knees until you are able to pop it, and peeling a banana using only your lips and tongue. Don't overdo it!

The most specific exercises involve, of course, the muscles specific to sex—your pubococcygeus muscles, the ones that anchor the base of the sexual organ in men and surround the sexual organ in women. In men and women these muscles allow control of what passes through the pee-pee tube—so you can give them a workout by squeezing off the flow. And you can pretend to squeeze off the flow even when you're not flowing. You can do these exercises in public, but remember that they draw less attention if you don't scrunch up your face at the same time you're scrunching up your pubococcygeus muscles. When these muscles are in shape, say the sexperts, everything gets better sexually, and, strengthening these muscles can also come in handy when you're peeing beside the car at the trailhead and another car suddenly pulls up.

FLEXIBILITY TRAINING

Everyone should be able to lean over and touch their toes, or at least their knees, in order to maintain enough flexibility to prevent damage to muscles and tendons during sex. In addition, becoming more flexible will allow you to attempt more fascinating things during sexual activity. Flexibility extremists reportedly can lean over and do what dogs do to their sexual organs, but some authorities question these reports. If you're interested in this and other interesting forms of sexual flexibility, it is strongly recommended that you use the Universal System of Sexually Unusual Contortions (USSUC), devised and made available by the friendly staff of the International Yoga Center for Sexual Looseness, founded by the Maharishi Beenderedundat. It is also recommended that you encourage your partner to stay flexible, too.

Mental Fitness for Fooling Around

Many people forget that the mind and the body are one. You can keep your body ready, but your mind can, on admittedly rare occasions, lose interest. Prayer and meditation are time-honored ways to keep your mind in shape. More recent mind-conditioning methods include biofeedback, psychotherapy, neurolinguistic programming, self-hypnosis, and listening to recordings of Dr. Ruth over and over. You may also consider packing an XXX-rated book on your next outdoor adventure (see Appendix 5: Suggested Reading).

Eating Right for Fooling Around

Eating every so often, in general, has been shown to promote important biological processes, such as breathing. But do not underrate the value of proper eating when getting in shape for sex in the outdoors. For one thing, the consumption of certain foods has been proven to encourage the urge to mess around (see Chapter 5: Preparation Be Fore Play). For another thing, the act of eating itself promotes the health of certain muscles useful in sex. Recommended getting-in-shape foods include but are not limited to chewy granola bars, new carrots, old celery, and bubblegum (with the wrapper still on). After gaining confidence, try eating a few unshelled Brazil nuts. Sucking an avocado out of a hole in its skin has also been recommended—as has peeling a banana using only your lips. Here are some more basics:

1. Take it easy on fats of all kinds. Fats clog arteries, and arteries carry blood to vital organs, if you know what I mean.

2. Eat lots of red meat, the tougher the better, and masticate as long as possible, swallowing the juices before swallowing the hunk of cow.

3. Drink lots of coffee. Although incompletely understood, studies show that a high intake of caffeine promotes sexual vitality— perhaps because it keeps you awake longer.

Finding an Outdoor Sex Partner

"Love is the answer; but while you're waiting for the answer, sex raises some pretty interesting questions."

—Woody Allen

Once the decision to start having sex in the outdoors is made, one may then have to decide with whom. The with-whom decision may be required because (1) you don't already have a partner; (2) your current partner is not interested in sex in the outdoors; or (3) you are not interested in having sex in the outdoors with your current partner. (*Note:* In case of "3," it might be a good idea to hide this book.)

Taking One with You

Although you can find one on the trail, and you can read about that after a few more paragraphs, your chances for sex in the outdoors are much higher if you hit the trail with a partner already tuned into and, more importantly, accepting of your sexual needs, desires, and weird idiosyncrasies. If you don't already have such a partner, you probably need a hell of lot more than this book to help you, but here, not necessarily in order of importance, are a few suggestions:

1. Take out a personal ad (full-page, four-color ads gets more attention) in local newspapers, state, or national outdoor magazines, or, if you're really desperate, a smut magazine.

2. Read the personal ads in local newspapers, state, or national outdoor magazines, or, if you're really desperate, a smut magazine.

3. Go online and become a member of one of those matchmaking sites. State your desires frankly, make up a name, and send a photo of John Cusack or Angelina Jolie instead of yourself.

4. Go to local bars where outdoor types hang out, wear outdoor clothing (for example, Patagonia®) with the manufacturer's logo prominently displayed, order a single-malt scotch neat, and leer.

5. Go to Sierra Club meetings (or meetings of any local environmental group), carry this book, and leer.

6. Take an outdoor instructor course, and size up the other students.

7. Become an outdoor instructor, and size up your students.

8. Visit the State Home for the Sexually Needy.

OPENING LINES

When trying to pick up a partner for sex in the outdoors, you never get a second chance to make a first impression. These opening lines have worked, occasionally, for some people. Remember to watch closely for the potential partner's reaction.

1. "My friends call me Studmuffin of the Mountains."

2. "Guess what I have that takes both hands to lift. *Hint:* It's not my backpack."

3. "That sport-bra would look great on my tent floor."

4. "I can see through your clothes."

5. "Let's go some place quiet and practice howling like coyotes."

6. "Would you like to see a photo of me wearing nothing but a climbing harness?"

7. "Have you ever sunburned your butt?"

8. "I'm not wearing any underwear."

9. "I got your name from a grateful search-and-rescue team."

10. "I don't mind if you sit on my face."

Finding One on the Trail

It is possible to find a partner for sex in the outdoors on the trail, especially if (1) you're having a really good day, and (2) you've been out for six months alone and so has he or she. Here are some ways to evaluate your chances:

1. If the other person passes you without making eye contact, rate your chances as slim or none.

2. If the other person stops and introduces herself or himself, your chances are a little better.

3. If the person who stops is wearing shorts that reveal a lot of leg, your chances are improving.

4. If the person who stops is wearing shorts that reveal a lot of bum or pubic hair, your chances are good.

5. If the person who stops is naked, your chances are really good.

6. If the person who stops is naked and it's winter, your chances are really, really good.

7. If the person who stops is naked and has a shoulder tattoo that says, "Just Do It," your chances are excellent.

8. If the person who stops is carrying a vibrator in one hand, your chances are very excellent.

9. If the person who stops is naked, tattooed, carrying a vibrator in both hands, and drooling, you're probably better off not making eye contact.

You can also size up a potential sex partner by closely observing subtle signals from her or his campsite. Things to watch for include:

1. Underwear drying on top of the tent or from the limb of a nearby tree. An okay signal.

2. Very skimpy underwear drying on top of the tent or from the limb of a nearby tree. A very okay signal.

3. Someone drying near the tent or tree. A good signal.

4. A vibrator lying on the ground near the tent. A very good signal.

5. A wet vibrator lying on the ground near the tent. An excellent signal.

6. A patch, sewed to the backpack, that reads "Outdoor Sex Club: Lifetime Member." A very excellent signal.

When the time comes to pop the question, your approach is, of course, entirely up to you. You can be blatantly open, subtly suggestive, teasingly cute, or charmingly assertive—whatever feels natural to you. You can also beg and grovel. You have nothing to lose but your reputation, dignity, and self-respect—and maybe a few teeth.

Preparation Be Fore Play

"An ounce of preparation is worth a pound of Blackberry Love Liquor."

—Benjamin Franklin Jones

In spontaneity may arguably arise the greatest source of enjoyment. There's nothing like a little well-planned spontaneity to improve sex in the outdoors. Remember the Six P's: Prior Planning Prevents Piss-Poor Performance. Forethought may prove almost as valuable as foreplay.

Geographical Route Finding

A lot of people who have sex in the outdoors don't know where they're coming. With thoughts of sex running rampant, they run rampant and lose track of the track and/or trail. That's a big reason why there are search-and-rescue teams. A well-laid plan to getting, well, laid includes planning a route. The route should include a few nice things to see (but not too many— you don't want distractions), pleasant camping spots, sources of fresh water, and a clear and easy path to follow. For reasons of privacy, good route finding should also include choosing a route that gives you the least possibility of seeing lots of other people—unless, of course, you're hoping to pick up a sex partner on the trail (see Chapter 4: Finding an Outdoor Sex Partner). A map and compass, or GPS unit, may be helpful (but usually not in picking up a sex partner). Although, if you do meet someone interesting, you can mark them as a waypoint on your GPS unit.

Sometimes your route of choice will require a shuttle. For instance, say you're rushing down a river, in a boat, or hiking a trail that doesn't end where it starts. When your trip is over, your car isn't there. So you arrange to have your car shuttled from the start to the finish. Understand? Okay, then consider hiring me to shuttle your car. For $10,000 I will shuttle any car anywhere in the United States. For $100,000 I will shuttle a car anywhere in the world. If you are considering hiring me, please follow these easy directions:

1. Send me the money.

2. Send me a map with directions to the exact location of your car, and a map with directions to the exact location you want your car to be—and when.

3. Send me the key or keys to your car.

4. Place another set of keys on top of the right rear tire, in case I lose the set you send.

5. Bury another set of keys 200 feet (70 adult paces) on a compass bearing of 69 degrees from the left-front corner of the bumper of your car, just to be safe. Dig deep enough to leave the keys in mineral soil.

6. Leave a set of keys on the front seat of the car. If all the other keys are unavailable, I can always break into your car.

7. Let me know if you want the car back in the same condition you left it in, or if you require the same car back.

Anatomical Route Finding

If you're new to sex, outdoors or indoors, your preparation should include a bit of research into the anatomy of the opposite sex. I will assume, at this point, that you're relatively familiar with your own anatomy and, therefore, the anatomy of other members of the same sex as you. If you prefer others just like you then you are way ahead of the game. There are plenty of books out there that will help you, but books with detailed pictures are more fun. *Opening Line to Avoid:* "Will you quit beating around the bush, George, and get to the point!" Once again, a map and compass may be helpful.

Equipment

When preparing for most outdoor trips, packing right means packing light. Who wants to waste a lot of valuable energy carrying too much weight? *Excuse to Avoid:* "Not tonight, Melvin, I'm just too tired!" Choose a small backpack. When it's full, a clear sign has been given that enough stuff has been packed. Distribution of gear between partners is significant, since weight bearing carries an importance of its own. Rubbing shoulders tired from the load of a pack often leads to rubbing more interesting body parts. Packing light may safely be ignored when planning many water-based adventures, but, don't forget, shoulders often need rubbing after a day of wielding a paddle, too. *Opening Line to Remember:* "I once took a course in massage therapy."

SHELTER

Lying out under the stars has a lot going for it if environmental conditions are favorable, but never leave civilization without a tent. Tents are insurance, providing protection from wind, rain, snow, sun, cold, insects, arachnids, and many species of wild mammals, including Peeping Toms. A candle lantern fills the fabric-walled bedroom with a soft, romantic glow. A well-placed campfire, when appropriate, flickers delightfully through the bright-colored nylon. Tarps give some insurance, but not enough. Carry a tent.

Choose a tent that sets up quickly and easily. Practice setting up a new tent at home to prevent frustration in case spontaneity raises its lurid, grinning face. How devastating to find the mood shattered by one's inability to fit the appropriate pole into the correct slot. But no matter how easily it sets up, always consider asking for assistance. Setting up the tent may be a shared experience that has a chance to provide a subtle basis for a later and decidedly more intimate shared experience.

Freestanding tents are obviously the best choice. They can be set up in almost any terrain, and there are no tight lines to fall over when you slip out for a pee. (*Note:* A self-deploying tent, like a self-inflating sleeping pad, is a terrific piece of gear, something wonderfully advantageous should a sudden urge strike.) And don't pick a tent that's too small. Plenty of room should be available for rolling around inside. When choosing a tent, consideration should be given to favored sexual positions. Who wants to be constrained by lack of space? On second thought, consider all sexual positions. Who wants to be constrained? Solo shelters are generally unacceptable unless, of course, you're alone and fully expect to stay that way. Huge base camp tents are okay for group sex (see Chapter 8: Variations on a Common Theme: An Environmental Perspective).

Sleeping Bags

Whoever came up with zip-together sleeping bags should be awarded the Nobel Prize for Outdoor Sex. Whoever travels into the outdoors with mismatched sleeping bags is not dedicated to achieving a maximal sexual experience. *Excuse to Avoid:* "Margaret, that cold draft turns me off!" For those who haven't noticed, the whole of the space within zip-together bags is greater than the sum of their individual spaces. *Excuse to Avoid:* "That won't work, Merv . . . there's not enough room!" In some cases, ending up with bags that zip together may require creative thinking: "OK, you bring the wine, and I'll bring the bags." Or: "Did you know I got *two* sleeping bags this year for Christmas? We might as well use them, and you can leave your old one at home."

The loft of the bags, which determines how much body heat they retain, should be appropriate to the season, but not too appropriate. If you anticipate sharing some heated moments, always opt for a bag with a little less loft than the expected ambient air temperature would indicate. *Opening Line to Remember:* "I think you'd be warm enough if we snuggled."

Sleeping Pads

Proper choice of sleeping pads rates at least as important, or perhaps even more critical than, the proper choice of sleeping bags. Standard air mattresses are simply too great a risk. They may deflate at the most inconvenient moment or, even worse, pop and eliminate all immediate hope for comfort. Old-fashioned outdoors folk may be heard extolling the acceptability of closed-cell foam pads. One thing all these old-fashioned types have in common is a failure to ever lie down on a self-inflating outdoor mattress. More up-to-date outdoor enthusiasts know that a couple of modern, rugged, self-inflating pads give a wide margin for safety as well as greater comfort while providing protection from rough, hard, cold ground. These, too, by the way, are available in models that attach to each other, insurance against a sudden shift in comfort.

The truly dedicated always carry a third pad, leaving out less essential items . . . such as, say, food. A third pad will serve one of two purposes: (1) It can pad the extra space in the tent for those who *really* roll around a lot, and (2) it can be added where pressure points exist, for example, under the hips, for extra warmth and comfort. *Excuse to Avoid:* "I'm sorry, Myrtle . . . I just can't find a comfortable position!" (*Note:* Fanatics have been known to carry *four* sleeping pads.) And, remember, despite the label "sleeping" pad (or "sleeping" bag, for that matter), whether one actually sleeps or not is another consideration altogether.

CLOTHING

Once upon a time outdoor clothing resulted exclusively from the weaving of natural fibers, and came in drab color choices of dark earthy tones. Clothing today consists primarily of long chains of petroleum molecules in colors described by long chains of fabulous words, for example, Tortugan Parrot-Feather, East African Sunset, Guatemalan Orchid. For the outdoor sexual enthusiast, the important considerations once were "Am I protected from the environment?" and "Will this stuff come off easily when I no longer want to be protected?" (*Note:* If things work out, and the other person is taking your clothing off you, your outdoor wear should be a challenge to remove but not a hardship.) Although these are still important points to consider, today the additional question is asked: "Do I look good?" This is not an inconsequential question if you have to get the attention of a potential partner. In many species, and increasingly so with humans, it is the "best dressed" individual that attracts the mate.

Confusion mounts as the customer must choose clothing to match the intended outdoor pursuit. So speaks the salesperson: "A pile sweater? Will you be backpacking, mountain biking, canoeing, rock-climbing, high altitude mountaineering, cross-country skiing, kayaking, or trying to pick up a date at the Boulder Mall?" *Excuse to Avoid:* "I like you, Martin, but your fuchsia Gore-Tex shorts clash with your scarlet Capilene one-piece longjohns!" Fortunately, the accepted dress for the sex act itself has changed little with the ages.

Food and Wine

Traditionally, an enjoyable meal has been a preface to well-planned sex. A few pre-trip questions about what the other person likes would certainly be appropriate, but here are several suggestions: (1) Choose foods that are politically correct—or at least acceptable by Greenpiece, the organization that sets standards for environmentally correct outdoor sex. Imagine opening a can of tuna to display parts of another dead fish that had been caught in a net! There goes your evening. (2) Choose foods from the category marked "aphrodisiac," foods such as dark chocolate (including green M&Ms), oysters, onions, tomatoes, cherries, cherry tomatoes, bananas, fish (including eels), broad beans—and did we mention chocolate? Season everything with hot spices—except the chocolate. (*Note:* Playing with your food, for example, hide-and-seek the cherry, can be a great way to break the ice.) (3) Don't eat too much. *Excuse to Avoid:* "I can't, Marge . . . I'm too full!" (4) Carry foods that can be licked off your partner, for example, jam, honey, syrup, whipped cream, artificial sweetener (for dieters), and bacon grease (for devoted carnivores). And lastly, (5) don't drink too much alcohol. A cup of wine heightens interest and mellows mood. Too much firewater and the water puts out the fire.

MONITORING ALCOHOL INTAKE

Contrary to what you may think, there are indications that you've had too much alcohol to drink. For instance, if you can't remember if your partner had an orgasm or not, you've probably had too much to drink. If you can't remember if you've had an orgasm or not, you've definitely had too much to drink. If you can't remember who your partner is, you've had *way* too much to drink. If you can't remember who you are, you should see a doctor . . . soon. If you've lost interest in having sex, you're an alcoholic. Puking is another bad sign—as well as being a disruption to the event.

Improvisation

One is limited only by one's imagination. No shelter? Crawl under some deadfall or into a cave. No sleeping pad? Rake some leaves and pine needles together. No sleeping bag? Use your clothes. No food? Go hungry. No one to have sex with? Go back to the start of this book, and read more carefully. In the spirit of our forefathers and foremothers, who challenged and tamed the outdoors, and who obviously had sex, do not be denied by the lack of a few amenities. Where there's a will, there's a way! *Excuse to Avoid:* "Oh no! I forgot the (fill in the blank)!"

Sexual Adjuncts

> *"Sometimes a cigar is just a cigar."*
>
> —SIGMUND FREUD

Here personal preference is the only guiding factor, but, remember, the ability to improvise (see p. 34) is one of the greatest signs of someone who is truly skilled in sex in the outdoors. Try humming, as one example, while performing oral sex, and you may never carry a vibrator again. Vegetable oil and the rubber gloves from your first-aid kit, as other examples, have many uses.

As far as medical adjuncts to sex go, what's on, or recently just passed behind, everybody's lips is a new drug similar to Viagra. You may be interested to note that the makers of this drug will soon be offering the drug in powdered form—suitable for mixing with alcoholic drinks—to be sold with the name Mount and Do. It will now be possible for a man on the trail to literally "pour himself a stiff one." It is anticipated that Mount and Do will give new meaning to old terms such as "cocktail," "highball," and "stiff drink."

Note: The long-term implications of use of this new drug in relation to certain medical procedures needs to be considered. Over the past few years, for instance, more money was spent on breast implants than was spent on Alzheimer's disease research. It is possible, therefore, that within the next 25 to 30 years there will be a large number of people hiking around with huge breasts or notable erections but who are unable to remember what to do with them. Caution is advised!

Special Techniques
for Special Places

*"It is during sex that our bodies do, or at least try to do, the most
magical and wonderful things. We grab and grope, slide and
squirm, reach and stretch, strain our muscles, and perform feats of
agility that would flabbergast an ape."*

—RICHARD SMITH,
IN *The Dieter's Guide to Weight Loss During Sex*

When the going gets tough, the intelligent go someplace else . . . where the
going isn't so tough. One of the greatest reasons, however, for the survival of
humans as a species is probably our ability to figure out how to make do with
situations when there simply aren't any immediate alternatives. "Special
Techniques for Special Places" is a celebration of human adaptability and
perseverance. One who successfully attempts to do "it" in a "special" place
does so for the obvious reason—which is, naturally, the chance to brag about
a heroic act performed against insurmountable odds under extremely adverse
conditions.

High Angle Sex

For those who enjoy the vertical world—finger jams, sewing-machine legs, desperate moves with poor protection—the term "safe sex" takes on a whole new meaning. First, as with all outdoor pursuits, choice of companions is the prime predictor of success. The climber must find an acceptable partner whose lead can be followed or who can follow the lead. What good are lofty thoughts of sex when you and the object of your desire end up separated by 165 feet of 11-millimeter Perlon? *Excuse to Avoid:* "Sorry, Elwood, this pitch won't go for me!"

Next, the climber must be very sure of the quality of the equipment he or she has chosen and the security of the anchors he or she has placed. Now clip in one of those tidy little nylon bedrooms, one that has a cover for privacy, the one that has been hanging all day in a haul bag at the end of the rope. Views tend to be grand, but are often best avoided (except for the up-close and personal views). The next move is the crux—getting out of harnesses, out of clothes, and back into harnesses without falling to an untimely-but-undoubtedly-much-publicized death. Before getting down to business, check to make sure you are both secured to tethers of a length appropriate to fulfill your high hopes. Hopefully, you are both wearing harnesses that won't get in the way . . . too much. Practice at home prior to attempts on a vertical face is strongly suggested. *Opening Line to Consider:* "Don't worry, Babe, I've done this before!"

Being, for the most part, afraid of heights, I have had to rely on first-hand accounts from friends who have a better sense of balance and less fear. My favorite story is from El Capitan's Salathe Wall, where the evening assault was on a noted female climber. During the act, he said, she had unbuckled the leg straps of her harness; and a shift in the hanging platform shoved her waistbelt up to her armpits. The deformation of her chest, she said, was alarming. I don't remember if they made the summit or not.

Laying While Belaying

For those who can't wait till bedtime, or who think the thrill would justify the risk, some belay points offer an opportunity for sex in the outdoors. Ledges are considered the most acceptable, but, hey, any port in a storm.

Discretion is advised. *Excuse to Avoid:* "You're not clipped in!" *Excuse to Accept:* "No way, Eleanor. If we botch this, we die!"

Once again, I turn to a friend of mine who claims that, in a rash act of spontaneity, nine months before the birth of her first child, she found love on a ledge, with several extremities hanging over the void, a most exhilarating experience.

Going Down Below Ground

The cave's a fine and private place, but few there are that there embrace. Caves offer the possibility of some advantages—silence, privacy, the dramatic echoes in an underground cavern. Most importantly, squirming through snug passageways has made you both horny, and there's nobody else around. Caves also provide some disadvantages. They are chilly, damp, dirty, and infinitely dark. "It is not the darkness I fear," whispered Elmer, "it is what the darkness hides." Comfortable dry bedding, a warm thermos of mulled wine, and adequate lighting may provide an opportunity for an unusual sexual experience. *Excuse to Avoid:* "I knew you were down there somewhere, Elsie, but I couldn't find you."

As with heights, I have no great fondness for caves, and I'm often heard echoing the words of the chronicler of old: "There is time enough for the earth in the grave." There is something weird, to my mind, about those people who go underground voluntarily before they are dead. My information comes from a caving instructor friend who claims to have been in many tight places in caves of the Midwest.

The Rush of Swift Water

Ever bounce along on a rubber raft through Class III and IV water, looking at the way some of the other scantily-clad rafters are bouncing along, feeling the warm sun put an itch in your britches? Ever wonder what it would be like to intimately share the bouncing? Like a waterbed, perhaps, but carried to a dare-devilish degree. Here are several suggestions: (1) Do not remove personal flotation devices (PFDs). (2) Do not try this without a third, understanding companion who is competent and willing to maintain control of the raft. (3) Do your part to keep the raft upright by striving to cooperate with the oarsperson and thrust yourself into the oncoming waves. You don't want to end up rolling in the haystacks. *Excuse to Avoid:* "I can't swim!"

I saw this first on the lower San Juan River of southeastern Utah. Magnificent sandstone edifices rose from both banks of the turbulent yellow water. A brilliant April sun warmly filled a soft blue sky. It was a large raft, and more than one understanding companion was ogling the act. I sat taking a break from paddling my canoe, stretched out on a riverside dune of white sand. As the raft flowed past, I realized what I was seeing and looked away . . . as soon as they were far enough downriver for the details to be lost through my binoculars.

Swamp Thing

Extensive marshy areas offer days of wandering narrow, wet passages through geographic regions without a single square foot of solid ground. Canoes are the only crafts small and maneuverable enough to allow access, while providing an acceptable-but-tippy base for overnighting. One learns to excrete body wastes while balanced delicately over the gunwale, to cook with the stove balanced delicately on a thwart, and to do other-but-more-satisfying things while balanced extremely delicately. *Here are some suggestions:* (1) Place unneeded gear in a waterproof bag, tie off the bag, and let it float beside the canoe during the night; (2) Keep your centers of gravity low, and (3) Plan shifts in position well in advance.

I remember one night in Florida, the moon almost full, a gentle breeze keeping the mosquitoes down while carrying the scents of sawgrass and palm, the chitter of night birds, and the bark of alligators. I wish I could say more, but that's all there is . . . I was alone. I wish I could brag of heroic acts performed against insurmountable odds under extremely adverse conditions.

Environmental Exposure

"Although nature and natural causes be forced and resisted ever so much, yet at last they will have their own way again."

—GEORGE BEST

Sex in the outdoors involves exposure of body parts—to a partner or two, in many instances, and to the environment, at least to some degree, in almost all instances. For that reason, a book on sex in the outdoors needs to cover, so to speak, those parts.

Cold

Few, if any, historians recognize the role cold has played in human evolution. Even in the hairiest moments of human pre-history, *Homo sapiens,* or something vaguely resembling that species, were never adequately prepared to deal with cold. When the earth started to cool down planet-wide, early humans were required to take the hairy skins from other species and wear them to make up for their own evolutionary inadequacies. To take hair from other pre-historic creatures necessitated, of course, the taking of their lives as well. (*Note:* Volunteerism never became very popular until the Republican

Party came along.) Not many people today realize that this was the original Cold War. Early humans also discovered a satisfaction that came from the act of killing, whether or not they needed hair, or food, and they passed that satisfaction on to all future generations. Thus, cold became the progenitor of all Regular Wars and murder, and, even now, humans speak of unkind fellow humans as being "cold-hearted" or "cold-blooded."

Millennia passed and humans learned other ways to help themselves survive in the cold. They learned, for instance, that lying around on the ground was not as warm as lying around on the hairy skins of other animals. So, beds were invented, another example of how cold has led to destruction of other life forms. The invention of beds soon led to the discovery that snuggling with another pre-human was warmer than sleeping alone. Snuggling naturally led to sex because the "act" produced lots more heat than simple snuggling. Thus, cold led directly to sex in the outdoors as a sport, rather than something done only to reproduce the species. Later it was discovered that other things improved sex in the outdoors, such as a roaring fire and strong wine, and, as a by-product, it was noted that fire and wine also helped one cope with the cold.

Humans who did not learn to cope with the cold died. It was said, once language was created, that they had died from "exposure" of the outside of their bodies to low temperatures. This was true until the 1950s when hypothermia—getting too cold on the inside of the body—was invented at a doctor's convention in New Orleans. The doctors were convening in New Orleans because physicians have historically had difficulty coping with cold, which is why hospital thermostats are always set around 100 degrees Fahrenheit. Undoubtedly, millions of people would have died from hypothermia if the thermometer had been invented sooner.

Today hypothermia ranks, understandably, as one of the greatest risks to the health and safety of those who pursue sex in the outdoors. It also ranks as one of the greatest deterrents to sex in the outdoors. Prevention is all-important. *Excuse to Avoid:* "No sirree! It's too cold!"

PREVENTION OF HYPOTHERMIA

1. SHELTER. To prevent hypothermia, some form of shelter is highly recommended. Originally, shelter meant a cave, and that still works today. In some regions, however, caves are hard to find, but tents are more than adequate (see Chapter 5: Preparation Be

Fore Play). It is best to secure a shelter before moving to the next step in prevention.

2. **FUEL FOR THE HUMAN ENGINE.** A quiet dinner for two is in order. Carbohydrates, tastefully spiced, burn more easily, providing quicker heat and energy. If this meal can be cooked and eaten within the heat of a campfire, hypothermia is prevented even more. If a campfire is inappropriate or impossible, at least have a candle.

3. **FLUIDS.** Although water works best as the fluid to drink for the prevention of hypothermia, wine should not be overlooked. First, the mellowing effect of the alcohol makes the human brain less aware of cold and, therefore, helps prevent excuses. Second, alcohol causes peripheral vasodilation, which is why skin gets warm and reddish. Vasodilated skin aids in the transfer of heat from the outside of the body to the inside, an important consideration in the prevention of hypothermia once snuggling begins. Furthermore, vasodilated skin has a heightened sensitivity to touch. *Opening line to remember:* "Just one drink, Suzanne. It helps prevent hypothermia!" (*Note:* Although wine is the traditional drink associated with sex in the outdoors, other forms of alcohol may work just as well.) Excessive consumption of alcohol is definitely not recommended, since it can destroy the mood as well as one's ability to find the tent.

4. **CLOTHING.** To prevent hypothermia, clothing should be loose-fitting and bulky. Loose-fitting in order to slip out of it quickly and easily so you're not over-exposed to the cold for very long. Bulky in order to stuff it around, under, or over you to hold in body heat. (*Note:* The key word to remember when dressing for the outdoors is "layering." Layering—and many people have forgotten this—originally meant "laying her," and it means today that you are dressed to allow for comfortable laying in a variety of climes.)

5. **PACING ON THE TRAIL.** Pacing is critical in hypothermia prevention for two reasons: (1) Overwork uses up energy stores, leaving you too exhausted to continue producing heat (as well as too exhausted to continue) and (2) Overwork makes you sweaty, and

you must stay dry to stay warm. *Note:* Sweating is acceptable, even recommended, once you have stopped humping the pack and started the other kind of humping.

6. ADJUSTING TO EXTREMES. Since the nature of sex in the outdoors inherently tends toward heat and sweat, allowances should be made for adjusting to these extremes. This is perhaps simpler than it sounds. When you feel yourself getting hot and sweaty, unzip the sleeping bags and throw off the excess coverings, i.e., bulky clothing. When you feel yourself getting chilled, zip up the bags and pull the excess coverings back over you.

Since hypothermia first and foremost reduces one's ability to think clearly, despite the most profound precautions, you may find yourself responsible for the care of a hypothermic companion. It may prove fortunate that sex in the outdoors, in addition to being a risk, has long been recognized as a treatment for hypothermia—which brings us to the next topic.

TREATMENT OF HYPOTHERMIA

1. ACTIVE EXTERNAL REWARMING. This is sometimes known as the Cuddle Technique. For maximum treatment, both parties should be naked and as much skin as possible on the normothermic person should be in contact with as much skin as possible on the hypothermic person. Don't forget that a cup of wine helps maximize skin-to-skin heat transfer. Both parties should be bundled in as much insulation as possible, including insulation from the cold ground, and care should be taken to make sure there are no leaks in the bundling where Cold Monsters can sneak in and take a bite. If zip-together sleeping bags are being used (a great advantage), a third normothermic person can be added to the treatment, but the third person should be someone you know really well.

2. ACTIVE INTERNAL REWARMING. This is sometimes known as the Copulation Technique. Follow the recommendations for Active External Rewarming with the addition of blatant sex. Care must be taken to monitor the patient for the Sexual Thermodynamic Reversal Phenomenon, which states that, physiologically, it is easier to cool down a human than to warm one up unless sex is added, and

then it is easier to warm up a human than to cool one down. In the case of the thermodynamically unstable human, this warming up process may produce excessive heat that could be a problem. It is strongly recommended that the care provider start slow and build gradually toward a climax of heat production.

Frostbite

Unlike hypothermia, in which the whole body gets cold, frostbite happens when the cold takes a bite out of a localized area of the body. During sex this happens because one's mind is somewhere else. It happens most often to toes that somehow ended up sticking out of the sleeping bag, or the butt, for the same reason. (*Note:* The expression "I froze my butt off!" originally came from a sexual experience near Gunnison, Colorado, in 1853, when Captain Gunnison's troops first encountered, simultaneously, extreme winter conditions and Ute maidens.) Other body parts can be involved, especially if you fall asleep exhausted and carelessly covered. Frostbitten parts can be recognized because they will be pale and numb . . . unlike the rest of the body. Treatment for frostbite should be immediate and gentle skin-to-skin contact. *Opening Line to Remember:* "It looks like frostbite to me, Bubba!"

Heat

Although the risk is low, it is generally accepted among the experts that certain predisposed individuals can become too hot—or hyperthermic—while having sex in the outdoors. At special risk would be those individuals who hadn't had "any" for a long, long time. Environmental conditions to consider avoiding, in order to prevent hyperthermia, would be direct sunlight when the ambient air temperature is high and the humidity is almost as high. For example, Florida during the daylight hours should be considered a high-risk region for sex in the outdoors, which is why there are more air-conditioned motel rooms than private homes in the Sunshine State. Hyperthermia should, however, be thought of as a serious threat to one's sex life, and treatment should be appropriate.

Treatment of Hyperthermia

Cooling off the patient is the only effective treatment. After moving the patient to a shady spot, remove all clothing, if this hasn't already been done. Fanning and massaging are effective means of cooling, especially if the patient's skin has been wet beforehand. If ice is available, it can be rubbed gently over the patient's skin, especially in areas of the body where ice is seldom rubbed. Care must be taken to avoid cooling the patient too rapidly, which has been known to produce heat.

Sunburn

A lot of direct sunshine produces more potential problems than just heat—ultraviolet radiation, for instance. It's the ultraviolet radiation (UVR) that causes sunburn. UVR takes time to burn human skin, so it probably won't mess up your first sex-in-the-sun experience. But if you're planning a multi-day outdoor trip, for example, beachcombing in Baja, you'll definitely want to take precautions in order to prevent Burned Buns Syndrome (BBS). BBS has been known to prevent sex.

Precautions to prevent sex-in-the-sun-burn before it prevents sex include but are not limited to: (1) Doing it in the shade, which is possible on many lakeshores and some beaches, especially if you bring your own shade, for example, a big umbrella; (2) Smearing a sunblock over everyone's entire body. Sunblocks let no UVR through, and include substances such as zinc oxide (ZO), which has the advantage of making you really slippery. *Warning:* Some people think being really slippery is *not* an advantage. ZO used to be available only in white, but now comes in brilliant colors. *Warning:* Some people find that a body entirely smeared with lime-green ZO is a turn-off; and (3) Coating everyone's body with a sunscreen. Sunscreens allow you to expose yourself to the sun longer without being burned. Every sunscreen container is labeled with a Sex Promotion Factor (SPF), which tells you how much longer you can have sex in the sun. A screen of SPF 15, for example, allows you to have sex in the sun 15 times longer than if you are not wearing that particular screen. Some sunscreens wash off easily with water or sweat, so be sure to ask for sex-proof sunscreen.

High Altitude Illness

It is a well-known fact that the higher one goes above sea level the less oxygen there is to breathe. This produces a condition known as hypoxia, which means low-oxygen. Hypoxia has a direct and immediate effect on the brain, causing it to have less fun, a serious consideration if one intends to have sex at high altitude. In addition to having less fun, other signs and symptoms of altitude illness include headache, nausea, loss of appetite, unusual fatigue, insomnia (not necessarily a problem), and lassitude (a condition describing loss of interest in sex, a serious problem).

PREVENTION OF HIGH ALTITUDE ILLNESS

1. ACCLIMATIZATION. This is the single most important factor in preventing high altitude problems. Acclimatization is a process in which the human body adjusts, and thus is able to function normally, under hypoxic conditions. Although it takes weeks for the full benefits of acclimatization to take effect, everyone should be able to function relatively normally after a couple of days at any given altitude. Since exercise tolerance will be lower, start slow . . . maybe with kissing and petting only on the first day. For individuals who are gaining altitude daily, i.e., high altitude mountaineers, it is strongly suggested that altitude be gained no faster than the body can acclimatize. There is a formula for figuring how fast altitude can be safely gained. It states that over 10,000 feet above sea level, no one should sleep more than 1,000 feet above their previous night's sleeping altitude. This does not mean that you can't gain more than 1,000 feet per day if you need, for instance, to ferry loads to a higher camp. It does mean that you should drop back down for the night. This is the source of the old mountaineering adage "Climb high, have sex low." *Excuse to Avoid:* "I'm sorry, Hank . . . I really do have a headache!"

2. FITNESS. Although fitness does not prevent altitude illness, it most definitely increases one's ability to acclimatize. If you are planning on having lots of sex at high altitude, you should obviously have lots at lower altitudes in preparation. *Opening Line to Remember:* "Honestly, Harriet, I need this in order to train for my next climb!"

3.DRINKING AND EATING. Drinking lots of water and eating lots of food helps prevent altitude illness. This, too, can be practiced at lower altitude.

TREATMENT FOR HIGH ALTITUDE ILLNESS

Descend, which, in this case, does not necessarily mean "go down."

THE PEAK EXPERIENCE CLUB

High altitude mountaineers who successfully attempt to have sex on the summit of the mountain they are climbing may qualify for membership in a small, prestigious, and little-known club. The summit must be higher than 14,000 feet above sea level, there must have been at least two climbers involved, and the one applying for membership must have had at least one orgasm. Send your name, the name of the mountain, and vivid details of the experience to The Peak Experience, P.O. Box 9, Pitkin, Colorado 81241. There is no financial cost for membership.

PHALLIC SHOCK

Although not a result of environmental exposure, and definitely not common, incidents of phallic shock are well documented, especially at high altitude, and should be considered before attempting sex. In phallic shock, the sudden rush of blood to the penis causes the victim to pass out. Treatment should include keeping the victim supine with his feet higher than his head (his hat-wearing head), and avoiding touching his penis. Prevention should include staying well-hydrated and letting things build up a bit slower. Deaths are rare.

Low Altitude Illness

This is sometimes referred to as drowning, a condition occurring when sex is attempted in water by those who are ill-prepared for the attempt. Here are some suggestions: (1) Practice at home in a bathtub first; (2) Fly to Hawaii or a lush Caribbean island for your first in-the-outdoors experience. The water will be warm (a plus), and salt water is more buoyant than freshwater (another plus); and (3) Wear a personal flotation device (PFD) or, better yet, snorkeling gear or, even better yet, SCUBA gear (but not a wetsuit).

Further precautions for freshwater sex include: (1) In shallow freshwater, the sex act is well-documented to attract leeches—leeches of the non-human variety. Their presence often alters the mood of the moment dramatically. And any freshwater that provides a home for ducks and snails may also be home for a schistosome that is deposited on the water's bottom in duck and snail poop. Thrashing around in shallow water can stir up the schistosomes, allowing them to take up residence on human skin, which causes a very uncomfortable dermatitis known as Swimming Sex-Itch. Keeping your freshwater sex in deep water will prevent the problems of leeches and itching; (2) In the Amazon River there lives a tiny fish that likes to swim up into and attach itself to human urethras. It works something like a heat-seeking missile. This problem, too, can be prevented by staying deep while having sex in the water.

Note: Reports from Alaska give evidence that it is possible to have sex in the water while wearing specially-designed wetsuits, but indications are that it is rarely worth the effort.

TREATMENT FOR LOW ALTITUDE ILLNESS

Prolonged mouth-to-mouth breathing interspersed with chest compressions at a ratio of 2 full breaths to 15 compressions is the treatment of choice for drowned persons. For maximum benefit, both mouth and chest should be bare. Mouth-to-mouth breathing should be practiced regularly at home and in the outdoors. Chest compressions should be practiced, but only pretend to compress the chest. Beware: This type of practice may be considered foreplay in non-professional circles. *Opening Line to Remember:* "Honest, Buffy, I need the practice."

Uninvited Guests and Other Dangerous Critters

It's a jungle out there, full of biters and stingers other than your sex partner. Some of those critters you'll want to know how to avoid.

INSECTS

One of the things that almost everyone who pursues sex in the outdoors desires is privacy. One of the things that insects deny is privacy. And there is a lot of exposure to insects during outdoor sex. "Hazel, is that you crawling up my leg?" All insects have three characteristics in common: (1) They all have segmented bodies; (2) They all have six legs; and (3) They all enjoy bothering humans. Many insects play an important role in the delicate balance of nature, but some do not. Take mosquitoes, for instance. There is absolutely no reason for a mosquito. Mosquitoes have ruined more outdoor sex than all other natural disasters combined. There are three ways to avoid contact with most insects:

1. Go to places where insects aren't. This is more difficult and costly than it sounds, but trips to the North and South Pole have been increasing in popularity over the past decade. It is reasonable to assume many of these trips have been planned in order to seek uninterrupted sex in the outdoors.

2. Make sure your tent has no rips in it and that the zipper works on the mosquito netting over the door. The rule is: Zip before you unzip. If you accidentally leave the tent door open too long, you might be better off keeping it open until all the insects, for example, mosquitoes, fly in, at which time you rush out and zip them up *inside* the tent, leaving you and your partner alone under the stars. *Note:* This requires perfect timing and is generally considered the second best plan.

3. Wear insex repellent. Insex repellent is any substance that repels insects while you're having sex. The newest innovation in a long line of insex repellents is a product that contains permethrin, which, when allowed to soak into clothing, actually kills insects when they try to crawl around on the clothing. The repellent, which is truly an insecticide, will not, say the experts, harm humans or dogs . . . but then the same words were once spoken about DDT. Permethrin will, obviously, not work, unless you are anticipating some well-clothed sex. Older products that contain DEET have been proven to repel insects. About a 30 percent concentration of DEET is all you need to repel all insects, and some arachnids, such as ticks. DEET must go on skin, and both partners must choose to wear DEET, because if only one opts for the repellent both end up wearing it anyway. Of course, liberal applications of lotions containing DEET can be fun and rewarding.

Totally ineffective as a repellent is a product called Skin-So-Soft—but it is harmless (to humans and insects), smells nice, and rubs on pleasantly. *Opening Line to Remember:* "You don't want to miss any spots, Hal. The 'skeeters 'round here are terrible!"

ARACHNIDS

Unlike insects, arachnids have eight legs and generally don't enjoy humans. Even ticks prefer mice and deer, and attach themselves to humans only when there is a shortage of other food sources. But, unlike most insects, the bites and stings of some arachnids can cause serious injury, devastating disease, and sometimes the death of sex in the outdoors.

TICKS

Ticks, worldwide, carry more diseases that humans can catch than anything except mosquitoes. They don't transmit disease by crawling around on human skin. They have to bury their heads and feed for awhile before germs are passed. It takes hours to days of feeding before enough germs are passed to make a human sick. Although some people seem to get quite sick when they find a tick creeping over their skin, that kind of sick doesn't count. Only fever, chills, nausea, achy joints, and rashes count. When ticks are discovered already buried in, they should be removed immediately. Many methods of tick removal fill the pages of medical history, and most of them have a common characteristic—they don't work very well. For instance, heating up a tick's rear end with a recently-extinguished match makes the tick very angry, causing the little guy or gal to expel lots of germs before backing out. Smearing a thick ointment over the tick allows feeding to go on for a long time before he or she needs to come up for air. Grabbing the tick and twisting it counterclockwise (or is it clockwise?) very effectively screws off the tick's head and leaves germs in the bitten person's body. This is what works: Use tweezers to gently grasp the tick near the patient's skin and slowly pull it straight out. In order to remove all ticks before germs are passed, it is necessary to perform careful tick-checks two or three times a day. Ticks prefer warm, moist, dark places on the human body, and tick-checks, as you might imagine, have led to much more interesting things. *Opening Line to Remember:* "Since you can't see down there, Boopy, I'll have to check it for you!"

SPIDERS

Where spiders are concerned, you especially want to avoid the *female black widow* (which may be brown, but has an hourglass-shape on the underside of her abdomen) and both sexes of the *brown recluse* (which may be black, but has a fiddle or violin-shape on the top of his or her head and back). Spiders normally roam around feeding at night, so stay in your tent as much as possible. Don't gather firewood in the dark, and don't wander outside barefoot or barebutt. Encounters with the fangs of these spiders are almost always painless, but excruciating pain comes within 15 minutes to an hour. The pain lasts a long time and effectively ruins the encounter you are after. Death is rare, so victims usually get to try again some other day. Leaving the outdoors to find a doctor is advised, but don't radio in the helicopter. Male humans, however, are often bitten on their testicles by black widows when the human uses an outhouse that the spider has chosen for a home. These victims may not get to try again some other day. Rapidly leaving the outdoors to find a doctor is strongly advised. Painkillers and sedatives may be given to the patient. Pouring cold water over the head of the frustrated sex partner is also recommended.

SCORPIONS

Scorpions, like spiders, generally shun the light of day, and anti-spider precautions will work for scorpions, too. Scorpions do not bite, but, instead, sting with the tip of their abdomen, which looks like a curled up tail. The sting of any scorpion is universally and immediately painful, but the only sting that may lead to a human death, in the United States, comes from a slim, yellowish- or greenish-colored resident of the desert Southwest. Scorpion stings are like a whopping bee sting, and the pain goes away fairly soon. Cold applied to the site of the sting makes the pain go away sooner. Pain may ruin the moment, but not necessarily the whole event. If the stung person, however, starts to feel sick and loses all interest in having sex, it is either (1) a result of the scorpion sting, or (2) a result of the atrocious smell from your polypropylene underwear combined with the unwashed condition of your body. In either case, you might as well leave the outdoors and seek help, a laundry, and a shower.

REPTILES

All snakes and most lizards should be considered dangerous, because so many people have been hurt running away from them. Running away, incidentally, is the appropriate response. Not all snakes are poisonous. The ones that are, in the United States, are either *pit vipers* or *coral snakes*. Pit vipers have slit, cat-like pupils and a heat-sensitive pit between eyes and nostrils. But if you're close enough to see that, you deserve to be bitten. Some pit vipers have rattles and some do not. Coral snakes have distinctly colored bands of red and yellow and black. "Red on black, venom lack, red on yellow, kill a fellow . . . or a woman." If you hear rattling, or see bands of bright color, or see a snake, or think a snake is nearby, run away. The only lizard in the U.S. considered poisonous is the *Gila monster,* which lives in a burrow in the Southwest near the dangerous scorpion. Gila monsters are black and orange and bumpy. Again, run away.

Reptiles are night-feeders and are seldom seen in the sunlight unless they are relaxing and working on their tans. Reptiles, by the way, can't roll over, which is why they are always pale and un-tanned on the bottom. Like humans, they do not enjoy being bothered when they are relaxing and tanning. If bitten by a poisonous reptile, stay very calm (ha ha), wash the wound, and casually leave the outdoors to find a doctor. Do not cut and suck, do not apply a tourniquet, do not apply a cold pack, and do not lick your car battery in an attempt to electrically discharge the venom. Those things don't work, and might cause significant harm. Consider carrying a product called a Sawyer Extractor, a suction device of proven worth for field removal of some venom. Suction devices can be of great value, especially if you're alone . . . and horny.

Large Mammals

Despite many interesting tales from the early days of the lonely mountain man who had sexual liaisons with large mammals other than humans, encounters with wild animals, especially carnivores, should be avoided. Bears, for instance, are capable, like many sex partners, of rapid and unpredictable mood changes. Bears are, furthermore, capable of removing significant body parts, and that would limit future sexual liaisons of any kind. If attacked, running away, in this case, is not recommended. Humans, in relation to other species, are remarkably slow. An exception to the do-not-run rule is this: When traveling in the outdoors with anyone who runs slower than you do, running away may be considered a viable option. If attacked by a black bear, say the experts, fight back. You won't win, but you may discourage the bear enough to save some of those significant body parts. If attacked by a grizzly bear, the experts continue, play dead. In most cases, you won't have to play very long because soon you'll be really, sincerely dead.

In hopes of preventing death-by-claw-and-fang, you may choose to:

1. Carry a very large gun or a small nuclear device. Neither of these will stop a ferocious carnivore, but both will allow you to blow off your own head before the ferocious carnivore eats it off.

2. Carry a can of bear repellent. This is an aerosol can of a fiery substance that burns the animal's eyes and mouth. The repellent should be sprayed all over your body shortly before the animal bites you.

3. Make lots of noise while in large mammal country. If you've ever felt like screaming while having sex, this would be a good time to let it out.

4. While camping overnight, hang all food and other carnivore-attractions, for example, toothpaste and strawberry-flavored sex oil, well off the ground. These procedures will not stop a hungry carnivore from figuring out how to get the food, but peanut butter tastes better than human and, while the animal is climbing the tree, you can run away.

5. As an alternative to Number 4, leave all the food on the ground and hang your tent between two trees at least 10 feet up in the air. This technique can give a whole new meaning to the expression "swinging," but be sure you're fully awake before slipping out to freshen up. *Note:* In fair weather, the "Swinging Method" also works with hammocks situated way up between two trees.

6. Travel in a group of four or more. Large mammals mistakenly think they cannot win if they attack groups of humans, and the group, if chosen wisely, might develop into some fascinating and slightly less dangerous liaisons.

7. Women who are having their period should sleep in the middle of the group. Men who are traveling with women who are having their period should sleep in the middle of the group. Women who are traveling with women who are having their period should sleep in the middle of the group. Everyone should have a large gun or a small nuclear device.

It should be noted that sexual myths surround several wild animals—unicorns, rhinos, and wood nymphs, for instance—and, for health and safety reasons, they should be recognized as false and misleading. Unicorns, for instance, will not cure ills, including pregnancy, when they touch someone with their horns. Neither do they impart sexual virility. The horns are, however, very sharp, and may leave a nasty wound. Rhino horns are, also, reputed to be of sexual value—not by touching them but by eating them. Many people, even today, consider rhino horns to be a powerful aphrodisiac. First, it doesn't work. Second, you have to chew a long, long time just to get one tiny bite down. Third, rhinos have to be killed to get their horns off, and rhinos have just as much right to life as you do. Furthermore, rhinos have just as much right to be horny as you do—maybe more so. *Note:* It is not known for sure whether it was unicorns or rhinos that left humans with the expression "horny." Wood nymphs, as well as water nymphs, flower nymphs, and dirt nymphs, were once thought to be the best sexual lovers on earth. It is now known that they are not, and, in fact, rhinos are slightly better.

Influential Plants

Many of the plants that grow outdoors are known for the mischievous pranks they play on humans. Over the centuries sex in the outdoors has resulted in quite a bit of contact between humans and plants. This contact varies from irritating to dangerous. On the irritating end of things, plant parts are always sneaking into clothing and bedding in the outdoors and producing scratchy interruptions in an otherwise pleasurable experience. Some plants are more than just irritating. Take the *stinging nettle,* for instance. Stinging nettles hang out near water, waving gently in an evening breeze, looking soft and inviting but waiting to sting and nettle. Some plants get carried away, producing effects that can be life-threatening. Even though it is assumed the plants mean no real harm, it remains in the best interest of all concerned to appreciate some of the pranks that might be played.

Poison ivy, as one example, likes to assume the appearance of an innocuous green leaf suitable for use as toilet paper. Once the oil of poison ivy (or oak or sumac) contacts your skin or clothing, it can be passed easily from one person to another through contact. Sex in the outdoors, therefore, may result in sharing more than was expected. Learn to recognize poison ivy, and lay down somewhere else. If contact has been made, immediately wash your entire body, the entire body of your companion, all your clothes, and anything else that could have contacted the plant. If someone starts to itch after washing, it means they didn't get washed soon enough, but it does not mean they still have the plant's oil on them. So it's okay to touch them. *Opening Line to Remember:* "Poor baby, let me scratch that for you!"

Deadly nightshade, an even more mischievous plant, grows bright red fruit all over the United States and seems to derive great mirth from pretending to be a huckleberry. People who eat the berry get a stomachache and throw up a lot. For some reason, many plants, including many domesticated vegetables, like to watch people vomit. As with all practical jokers, deadly nightshade needs to be careful. Before the berry ripens, it contains enough poison to kill an adult human. People who eat deadly nightshade get dry skin, blurred vision, hallucinations, convulsions, and a high fever. The old symptomatic saying goes like this: "Dry as a bone, blind as a bat, crazy as a loon, and hot as hell." Although that may describe some of your earlier sexual encounters, it is, where plants are concerned, not to be desired.

Pokeweed, sometimes called pokeberry, or just poke, is predominantly an Eastern plant that tries to trick the sexually-inclined with its name. *Warning:* Consumption of pokeweed has absolutely no effect on "poking." Pokeweed can, however, be safely eaten if the leaves are boiled, the water poured off, and the leaves re-boiled. Eating undercooked pokeweed causes a burning sensation in the mouth and throat, nausea, and stomach pain. Gastronomically speaking, you might as well pack in some freeze-dried lettuce.

Twenty-one species of *mushroom* contain the hallucinogens psilocin and psilocybin. Hallucinogenic mushrooms have been used for thousands of years to improve sex, and were known to the Aztecs as "the flesh of the gods." Psilocybin is a relative of LSD and has some of the same effects on the human brain: mood elevation and alterations in sensation. This can be really useful if you end up with someone who isn't much fun to be with. Hallucinogenic mushrooms should be considered tricky for three reasons: (1) They are illegal in some places, so you can get into real trouble; (2) They may look very much like some poisonous mushrooms and, if you eat a poisonous one by mistake, can get you into real trouble; and (3) They can give you a "bad trip" during which you might say and do things you regret later, which can get you into real trouble.

Climatic Concerns (Weather or Not to Do It)

Weather is well documented to have an impact on sex in the outdoors. Knowing what kind of impact, and how to take advantage of it, may prove of inestimable value.

Rain and Snow

The first thing to beware of is clouds. Clouds are water droplets gathering together. If water droplets clump up enough for gravity to have an effect on them, they fall as either rain or snow. Neither rain nor snow should dampen your experience. It is a proven fact that both rain and snow increase the chance you will have sex in the outdoors. It could be related to the seductive pitter-patter of rain, or the need to feel warmer, or hormone production increasing due to atmospheric pressure changes, or I could be making all this up. But rain or snow are always good reasons to set up the tent.

And, for emergencies, consider carrying a cagoule (also known as a poncho), the largest one you can find. Cagoules were once popular as outdoor wear, but have, in recent years, fallen out of fashion. A cagoule is an article of clothing that is more like a small waterproof tent than a raincoat. Although there is only one head-hole in a cagoule, there is often enough room inside for two people. Cagoules also block wind. For minimum impact, choose a color that blends in with the natural surroundings

Lightning

The ultimate culmination of clouds and wind is, of course, a storm. In warmer months, storms may produce the greatest climatic danger to those involved in climactic pursuits—lightning. Lightning is a massive discharge of electricity directed along the path of least resistance toward the nearest object, for example, tall things, or things standing alone in open spaces. It can hurt you in several ways: (1) Direct strike, in which case the victim becomes an overdone potato chip, and sex is completely out of the question forever more. *Note:* It has been suggested by sexperts that a direct strike may mimic the world's largest orgasm, but no one will ever know for sure;

(2) Splash from a nearby direct strike, in which case the victim can be burned or killed. *Note:* Survivors of splash incidents give a variety of sensory reports, none of which support the premise of the "Note" from Number 1 (see p. 59); and (3) Ground current, in which case the electrical current, running through the ground under the victim, may cause no more than a tickle, or may short the victim out totally. *Note:* Leg-to-leg ground current has some interesting theoretical possibilities for jump-starting people who are impotent. It worked on Frankenstein, didn't it? Stodgy research ethics committees have precluded further investigation into this area.

Close contact with lightning during sex should be avoided. It is unnecessary, if you know what you're doing, and it may be fatally dangerous. Avoidance can be achieved in several ways: (1) Stay off or leave mountains and ridges. Even moving a short distance may save your life. Lightning storms are *not* the time to try for The Peak Experience Club; (2) Stay away from bodies of water. Other bodies are okay; and (3) Stay away from single trees. Married trees are okay—or, at least, trees that are deeply committed to each other. In fact, a forest is a relatively safe place. (4) Stay out of shallow caves and overhangs. Deep caves are okay, if they are dry, but don't touch the walls during a storm. It's actually better if you don't touch the ceiling or floor either. Try hovering. (5) Stay out of open areas where you might be the tallest thing around. Putting your partner on top does *not* help. Lightning, in its dedication to reach the ground, will pass through both of you. (6) Always travel in the outdoors with someone who is taller than you are. And don't let them near you during the storm. *Opening Line to Beware Of:* "Oh, Sam, you give me a real tingle!"

If you are caught in a lightning storm, crouch. Crouch on your sleeping pad, if possible, to minimize conductivity. "Crouching" is an outdoor sexual position developed by the nomadic people of the Mongolian steppes where lightning storms are frequent. No illustrations are available at this time, but you can use your imagination. If you are in your tent when the storm hits, you can, of course, crouch inside your tent. History buffs may be aware that Genghis Khan was crouching in his tent at the time of his death—but no one knows for sure if a lightning storm was in progress outside his tent or not. It cannot be definitively stated, therefore, that crouching during a storm will save your life. It does promise, however, to make your last moments happier. *Opening Line to Remember:* "Don't be silly, Sally, this is only for your safety!"

Variations on a Common Theme:
An Environmental Perspective

*"Don't turn away from possible futures before you're certain you
don't have anything to learn from them."*

—RICHARD BACH IN *Illusions*

Bestiality

*"My schoolmates would make love to anything that moved, but I
never saw any reason to limit myself."*

—EMO PHILIPS

Many people mistakenly think "bestiality" means having sex *with* beasts
other than humans when, in truth, its historic meaning relates to having sex
like beasts other than humans. The practice of bestiality obviously dates
from long, long ago, when humans, relative newcomers to the animal world,

watched other animals having sex in order to learn how to do it. Bestiality is limited almost entirely to mimicking fur-bearing mammals, with the exception of a few reptiles. Mimicking bird-sex, for instance, is almost too ridiculous to even imagine. For one thing, birds aren't physically equipped with the same general type of sex organs as humans. And, for another thing, many birds have sex while flying in the air, and it's over really, really fast. Bees are even more boring, and whoever came up with the term "the birds and the bees" as an expression for having sex was singularly unimaginative.

Note: It might be possible for skydivers to have sex while falling through the air if (1) they started at a very high distance above the ground, and (2) they added a new dimension to the term "quickie." It is not known if this has ever been achieved . . . or even if it has ever been attempted. It would be so very greatly appreciated if anyone with knowledge concerning skydiving-sex would contact the publisher of this book with graphic details. Another volume in this exciting and enlightening series is anticipated. Names will be excluded at the request of anyone providing information. Thank you very much.

THE HISTORY OF BESTIALITY

There was a time, relatively long ago, when "bestiality" did mean having sex with beasts other than other humans. There are several reasons why the meaning changed: (1) With large mammals, and some reptiles, it proved very dangerous; (2) With the growth of the animal rights movement, it became increasingly important to show respect for wild animals. The rule of "Only Between Consenting Adults," once applied to animals other than humans, was terrifically difficult to honor, what with the language and cultural barriers. It was so hard, in other words, to know if you had the animal's consent; (3) With the increase in concern about practicing safe sex, it proved mighty difficult to know for sure if your would-be partner was carrying any disease that could be transmitted to a human; and (4) practically speaking, it was virtually impossible to establish the rapport necessary for a mutually satisfying experience.

Although it is possible for humans to have human-sex underwater (see Chapter 6: Special Techniques for Special Places), there would be no point in attempting to mimic fish-sex since they never even touch each other. Dog-sex was probably one of the first ones copied by early humans, since dog's tongues hang out and it looks sort of like they're having fun. Bestiality is practiced by most humans a little bit, but it doesn't take long for humans to move on to other forms of sex, since beasts other than humans are not very creative about doing "it."

Voyeurism

"A picture is worth a thousand words."

—ANONYMOUS

To differentiate between "bestiality" and "voyeurism," the former means, as mentioned above, mimicking beasts other than humans having sex, while the latter means just watching sex happening. Voyeurism, on one hand, may often lead to bestiality, since voyeurism-in-the-outdoors is, for the most part, a trans-species form of voyeurism. On the other hand, so to speak, voyeurism may provide incentive for masturbation (see p. 69). For people with a third hand, it can be a sexual variation all its own. Furthermore, voyeurism needs to be distinguished from watching dirty movies. Watching dirty movies or erotic scenes from *Wild Kingdom* does *not* qualify one as a voyeur, because to qualify requires watching it in the flesh or fur.

Society, in general, looks with disgust upon voyeurism, especially as it is practiced in the city. Anyone who spends much time in the outdoors knows that it is almost impossible to not practice trans-species voyeurism, at least to some extent, and those people should not feel like a lesser person just because they stopped and stared. (*Note:* It is possible to be outdoors a long time and *not* have a chance to participate in trans-species voyeurism, say, for instance, in the northern latitudes in winter . . . unless you are a dogsledder.) If you're out for a hike or a paddle, and you happen to stumble upon a couple of wild animals attempting to reproduce their species, and it embarrasses you, you can always turn away and pretend you didn't see. But do not underestimate the stage-setting value of trans-species voyeurism. If you can afford to be a little more liberal, try pointing and saying: "Would you look at that!" Such liberalism might help set a subtle yet pervasive tone for the outdoor trip, and who knows what that could lead to. *Opening Line to Remember:* "Gee, Ellie, do you think it's possible for humans to do what those kangaroos were doing?"

Just in case there are no muskrats or elephants messing around for you to ogle as a prelude to other sexual encounters, a bit of research may still allow you the opportunity to utilize trans-species voyeurism. While the wine bottle is being passed around the campfire, you can liven up the conversation (and, maybe, redirect a few thoughts) by storing some information beforehand and dropping it casually into the chatter: "Oh, by the way, did you know that geese mate for life, but mallards, when the urge strikes them, participate in a ducky form of hectic group love." Or: "Have you heard that dragonflies have sex on the wing, the female swinging like a trapeze artist below the male?" (For more information, refer to Mark Jerome Walter's *Courtship in the Animal Kingdom* or, even more revealing, Robert A. Wallace's *How They Do It*.)

Note: A few fortunate people actually walk up on two or more humans having sex in the outdoors . If they're truly fortunate, the humans having sex don't notice the voyeur, and he or she gets to watch for a while. These can be special moments and, if you're one of the truly, truly fortunate ones, you might qualify to have your story published in the *Voyeur's Yearbook*.

Ropes and Knots

"It's been so long since I made love I can't even remember who gets tied up!"

—JOAN RIVERS

French people, who are reportedly very skilled at sex in the outdoors, call roping *ligottage,* but over here in America it's usually referred to as "bondage." Bondage is the art of tying up your partner before having sex, a useful skill in the really old days when unwilling partners were common and perpetuation of the species was critical. Nowadays humans have done just about all the perpetuating they need to, and bondage has become a kinky variation practiced by willing partners. (*Note:* The kinks are in the mind, and should not be in the ropes.) The game of bondage takes a little practice so you don't screw it up, so to speak, and either waste a lot of energy you'll need later or else hurt someone.

First, it is important to work out a signal in advance in case it isn't fun anymore. Yelling and screaming, for instance, might be signs of fun or they might be signs of real distress. Hand signals don't work, of course, and code words are often useless since the tied-up person is often gagged as well. A good signal is one that can be hummed, such as, say, the opening stanza from *The Sound of Music:* "The hills are alive with the sound of music." Profuse bleeding and unconsciousness are also both pretty good signals that the fun has gone too far.

OUTDOOR BONDAGE SAFETY CODE

1. Everyone involved must agree beforehand and sign their name and the date on the dotted line below.

2. Nothing may ever be tied around anyone's neck.

3. Nothing may ever be stuffed into anyone's mouth other than things agreed upon beforehand.

4. Nobody may ever be left alone while in bondage.

5. All knots must be quick-release.

6. Everyone involved must promise to never tell.

Next, some rope or cord is needed, and outdoor trips usually have enough of that around somewhere. On climbing trips, seat harnesses and carabineers could be put into use. Bondage games are best played early in an expedition into the outdoors so the rope burns have a chance to heal before the return home. Slings from the first-aid kit work well, and, since they're soft, they probably won't burn as much. Slip knots are the preferred knot because they can be undone quickly if you hear somebody coming down the trail, or if you notice that your partner's hands or feet have become grossly swollen or blue. In extreme situations, tape or glue might work. Blindfolds should be considered if you or your partner are ugly.

Federal law requires that the Outdoor Bondage Safety Code be displayed prominently before the game of bondage can be legally played. A printed copy of this code, in a waterproof cover, can be ordered from the U.S. Department of the Interior, Washington, D.C., or you can make your own. *Excuse to Avoid:* "I'm sorry, Igor, but you haven't posted the code!"

Group Sex

"The closest I ever came to a ménage à trois *was dating a schizophrenic."*

—RITA RUDNER

When a group gets involved in sex in the outdoors, it's usually a group of men, although more and more groups of women are starting to acquire a taste for this activity (which may be one explanation for the proliferation of "women only" outdoor trips). Occasionally, in more liberated outdoor circles, both men and women are participating in group sex. In most cases, outdoor group sex starts around a campfire, after the evening meal has been prepared and eaten, when everyone is tired but not quite ready for the sack. A common group sex scenario sounds something like this:

FIRST SPEAKER: "Hey, did you see the boobs on that babe who passed us on the trail, the one wearing that little yellow sport bra?"

SECOND SPEAKER: "Gee, did I ever! I'd sure like to take a nap on that pillow!"

THIRD SPEAKER: "Nap!" Are you kidding? What I'd like to do is . . ."

And so the evening runs on until everyone, too tuckered out to continue, goes off to their respective sleeping bags. This is not a very high-grade form of sex in the outdoors, but, being almost as old as the "deed" itself, it is undoubtedly here to stay.

On rare occasions, group sex goes beyond the verbal stage. In this case, it is especially important to maintain group safety. As the old outdoor sex adage states: "The safety of the many outweighs the safety of the few." Special considerations for active group sex in the outdoors should include but are not limited to:

1. In cold environments, consider the "be like a bee" guideline. Bees, in winter, keep rotating so the warm inside bees change places regularly with the cold outside bees.

2. In hot environments, consider reversing the "be like a bee" guideline, and periodically have someone throw a pot of cold water into the center of the group.

3. In high-angle environments, be sure to check the sheer and tensile strength ratings of the ropes before going hog wild. The Canadian Bureau of Outdoor Sex Standards (CBOSS) has performed exhaustive tests on all brands of climbing rope available in North America. (*Note:* The Bureau is a little hard to track down. At this writing, they may be contacted at: CBOSS, General Delivery, Whitehorse, Yukon Territory.) It is strongly advised to keep one member of the group segregated and in charge of rope management in order to prevent entanglements that could otherwise last a lifetime.

4. On whitewater trips, special buoyancy considerations are required. As a rule of thumb, take the capacity rating of your craft and subtract two for normal group sex, and divide in half for really athletic group sex. Depending on your group, you may wish to round down to achieve an even whole number. Never round up. (*Note:* These rules do *not* apply to canoes.)

5. For in-the-ocean group sex, everyone should be required to wear a personal flotation device (PFD). It is recommended that you use the buddy-body system with periodic head counts to ensure that no one has sunk in the confusion. Use of shark repellent is optional but advisable.

Masturbation

*"I remember the first time I had sex. It was very frightening.
I was all alone."*

—Rodney Dangerfield

Masturbation, the skill of holding your own in the wilderness, was once considered a basic piece of knowledge, such as building a fire by rubbing sticks together, something essential to survival. But it is rapidly becoming a lost art. Nowadays, with the growing diversity of pornographic magazines and X-rated movies, the sophistication of vibrators, the availability of K-Y Jelly, and other technological advances, the old hand skills are being forgotten. With the modern back-to-nature movement, and its concomitant resurgence of interest in sex in the outdoors, perhaps there will be a renewal of interest in the preservation of some of the grand old ways. Let's hope so.

Anal Sex

Other than poor anatomical route-finding skills (see Chapter 5: Preparation Be Fore Play), the "other" orifice is sometimes used for several reasons: It's nasty, naughty, and, for some, nice. If taking a trip down the dirt road is your thing, don't let the great outdoors get in your way. If you're not a fan of the chocolate highway, a deep woodsy setting might just be the trick. This activity is very tiring, so have a snack beforehand. You don't want to embarrass yourself by bottoming out on your partner. And remember, however, that it's okay to be anally compulsive but not anally retentive.

Sexual Adjuncts Found in Nature

"To know when you have enough is to be immune from disgrace."
—LAO TZU

The use of objects found in nature to help satisfy you or your partner's sexual desires is limited only by your imagination—see Chapter 5: Preparation Be Fore Play—and a few rules. You're on your own with the imagination part, but here are the rules:

1. Your choice of nature's offerings should be agreed upon beforehand by all parties concerned. Believe it or not, some folks don't like the feel of salamanders.

2. Living flora are generally more accepting of a role as a sexual device than living fauna. Consider how a rabbit feels about being used in cancer research.

3. You don't have to negotiate with dead objects, but you should respect them.

4. There are soft pinecones and there are hard pinecones. There are small pinecones and there are large pinecones. Be careful!

5. Know your mushrooms well.

6. Cockleburrs, and other prickly plants, are out . . . regardless of their names.

7. Feathers are in, especially if they are no longer attached to the bird . . . unless it's a very sexy bird.

Some herbs found in nature have been used for centuries to enhance the sexual experience. These, in case you've forgotten, are known as *aphrodisiacs*. If you're hiking around in Mexico or the southwestern United States, for instance, keep an eye peeled for damiana, *Turnera aphrodisiaca,* well known for its aphrodisiac effect. About one hour before sex, make a strong infusion of the herb by steeping approximately 4,000 damiana leaves in approximately 18 gallons of boiling water for 10 minutes. When the water has cooled, soak in it until you're ready for intercourse. It gently stimulates the genito-urinary region. If you're in a hurry, or without an 18-gallon container, make a cup of damiana tea and drink it. It might work. If you're not in a hurry, try the recipe recommended by Dr. Cynthia Mervis Watson in her delightful book *Love Potions: The Doctor's Guide to Aphrodisia*. Soak about an ounce of dried damiana leaves in a pint of vodka for five days. If the vodka-damiana combo fails to work, at least you won't care as much.

Other naturally occurring aphrodisiacs include wild yams (another native of Mexico), saw palmetto berries, licorice root, ginkgo, sarsaparilla, kola nuts, red clover, and bee pollen. For recipes contact the Institute for Better Living Outdoors at (800) 555-5555 or (www.IBLO.org).

Outdoor Sex Etiquette

*"If you can't say something nice, don't say anything at all. If you
can't do something nice, don't do anything at all."*

—Ms. Manners

Etiquette, for those who have forgotten, means acting in a certain way
because it's the nice way to act and not because you have to act that way.
Law, for instance, says no one can kill Bambi unless it's deer season and a
license to kill has been purchased. Etiquette, on the other hand, says no one
should set their tent up in a bed of wildflowers because someone else might
come along later and be disappointed by a ruined flowerbed.

Minimum Impact

Sex in the outdoors undertaken by the incautious or ignorant can potentially
have a severe impact on an otherwise pristine wilderness area (see Chapter 2:
Why Have Sex in the Outdoors?). First, consider the visual impact. Imagine
the consternation of an insensitive (and undoubtedly undersexed and, thus,
unhappy) prude who comes walking over a ridge and sees the natural wonder of a magnificent vista blotted by a couple of people having sex in a high
alpine meadow! Instead, move into some bushes or into a stand of thick

timber, out of the open and well away from trails. Above the tree line, hiding among boulders should do. In the sandstone country of the high desert Southwest, there are neat little overhangs that conceal shady hidey-holes everywhere.

Lots of thrashing around in the same spot is bound to have a noticeable impact on the earth—crushed grass and compacted soil, for example—and is easy to avoid. Among trees the ground is covered with duff, a dense layer of decayed matter such as leaves and pine needles, and duff is relatively soft and comfortable and easy to restore after being thrashed around on. In the woods of the deep South, it is clearly understood that "moss be mo' bettah" . . . but watch out for the chiggers. Beaches and other sandy spots work well, too. Sometimes, even in summer, patches of snow can be found in the high country, and, if enough insulation is available, that makes a good place to indulge without much impact on the environment. Without adequate insulation, sex in snow can be a challenge, but so what?—nothing risked, nothing gained (see Chapter 7: Environmental Exposure).

Sound, too, can have a negative impact in an outdoor setting. Yells and moans will carry long distances over open water and across lush, wide meadows. Those same noises will disperse quickly among trees. Boom boxes are simply unacceptable in wilderness areas. If music is essential to your sexual experience, memorize the lyrics from *Man of La Mancha*—and sing. What you lack in accompaniment (or talent), you can make up for with gusto.

Natural water sources need to be protected. If you need to wash up— before or after—you can get by with jumping into a lake or wading into a stream or river. Soap, however, can be fun, but it should only be used well away from water sources. Here is the way to use soap for minimum impact. Everyone takes off all their clothes and gets wet in the lake or stream and fills all the available empty containers with water. Move about 200 feet away from the water source. Everybody lathers everybody else up really good, being careful to get the hard-to-reach places, and pours the water from the containers over each other. This is usually pretty noisy, so it would be best if you're in a stand of timber . . . where there's duff . . . and other people can't see you. *Opening Line to Remember:* "Let me scrub your back for you, Helen!"

Trash is ugly and should be collected before leaving the sex site. Check carefully for anything that could have been carelessly thrown aside in a moment of passion. Condoms can kill! A pelagic seabird washed up on the beach after becoming fatally entangled in a carelessly discarded sport-bra is a sad sight indeed! If you packed it in, pack it out. Fluff up the duff, smooth out the sand, wipe off the rocks, and so forth. The key to minimum impact is this: Make it look as though you never came.

Campground Etiquette

Not everyone will want to have sex in the outdoors way out in the wilderness. For owners of RVs, for instance (admittedly a tangential group of outdoor sex enthusiasts), the rules of etiquette are to keep the curtains closed, the door shut, and the shock absorbers in good repair. Campground tent campers should keep the noise down and the tent flaps closed. The general rule is this: Be sensitive to others less fortunate than you.

And consider the little children that so often litter campgrounds. Imagine them seeing something like a couple coupling. They might have boring parents who don't think sex in the outdoors is okay—and you might find yourself explaining or faking an apology to a red-faced mother or a red-necked father.

Note: In developing countries, tents are a novelty that often attract attention. I awoke in a tent in Belize once with a mass of little brown eyes peering through the mesh door. Gee, I was glad I wasn't having sex at the time . . . sort of.

Miscellaneous Considerations

If kids are members of the party you're traveling in the outdoors with, you probably (1) should plan on not having sex or (2) should bring a separate tent for the kids. If the kids are teenagers or, even worse, you agreed to chaperone a group of teenagers on a camping trip, it probably won't matter in the least that you have a separate tent. In case of teenagers, bear repellent works well . . . much better than on bears. Do not play dead. They just get more excited. Fighting back is probably the best plan.

If you end up with an overpowering urge to have sex with your partner, and you happen to be sharing a tent with another couple, the time has come for some frank talk. For any number of reasons, sharing a tent with a couple who is having sex may be acceptable. Etiquette requires, however, that you bring the matter up for discussion before other things get brought up.

Safe Sex in the Outdoors

"Be a virus, see the world."

—Gary Larson

Anyone having sex in the outdoors, or sex anywhere for that matter, who is not concerned about safety is either morally and ethically blind or stupid . . . or both. There are three areas of safety that need to be addressed: (1) Environmental safety. Cold can kill!; (2) Safety from disease. Nasty, microscopic life forms can kill!; and (3) Safety from getting pregnant. A woman who believes a man who said he'd had a vasectomy and it turns out he lied in order to talk her into having sex without birth control and she gets pregnant, can kill!

Environmental Safety

This topic has been dealt with in preceding sections of this book (see Chapter 7: Environmental Exposure).

Safety from Disease

Alone at last? Maybe not! Consider for a moment that delightful-looking partner on the other side of the tent, the one slipping into (or out of) something a little more comfortable. He or she could be infested with microscopic critters itching to head out on a trip of their own.

There are several ways to prevent the spread of disease through sex. One is total abstinence from sex, an undertaking that is, of course, totally out of the question. Well, maybe not totally. As far as I can tell from an exhaustive search of the literature on the subject, abstinence is acceptable for one reason: You're dead.

Another way to prevent the spread of disease is by taking universal precautions. To take universal precautions requires you to ask your partner: "Is there any disease in the whole universe that I could catch by having sex with you?" And your partner says: "No!" And you say: "OK, fine." Sometimes taking universal precautions does not work because some people will say anything in order to have sex. If one does not trust universal precautions, then one may resort to regional precautions. To apply regional precautions requires the use of a mask over the region of your mouth and nose and, if a male is involved, the use of a condom over the region where condoms are designed to go. *Note:* In the event that spontaneity or poor pre-planning finds you ill-prepared, regional precautions can be improvised by using plastic bags from your backcountry kitchen kit or rubber gloves from your outdoor first aid kit. As Einstein said: "Imagination is more important than knowledge."

The greatest threat to one's well being is undoubtedly a case of the Accidentally-Induced Death Sentence (AIDS). *AIDS* is a disease characterized by progressive deterioration of one's immunological system, leading ultimately to death from all the germs of the world that can no longer be fought off by the deteriorated immunological system. It is an unpleasant way to die and, since no one would choose it on purpose as an option, it is a syndrome described understandably but somewhat deficiently via the term "accidental." It is a popular theory that the AIDS virus, known as HIV (human immunodeficiency virus), and humans share a common ancestry, both having developed from the monkey population of Africa's wilderness. Or perhaps you prefer the theory that lets monkeys off the hook but skewers the World Health Organization (WHO) for mucking around with the smallpox vaccine. In either case, there are several ways to get AIDS, but the one of immediate concern is acquiring it from unsafe sex. HIV is carried in human blood and in human body fluids that make sex slippery. HIV is adaptable and found everywhere, from the hustle and bustle of big cities to the untrammeled forests of the earth's wildest land. The transmission of HIV can be prevented most effectively by using universal precautions against receiving this most unwelcome visitor into the inner sanctum of your body. *Excuse to Accept:* "We should be careful, Winona. I'm not well!"

Hepatitis B ("B" for Bad) is another potentially fatal disease that can be contracted while having sex. It's more common than AIDS, but, unlike AIDS, there is a very effective vaccine against hepatitis B. It takes six months for the vaccine to become completely effective, requiring safe summer frolics in the outdoors to be planned and prepared for around Christmas. As with condoms, wetsuits and tarps also provide some protection against hepatitis B and AIDS, but the sensory deprivation is astounding.

For those who are particularly fond of sex on the beach, a watchful eye should be kept open for *crabs*. Crabs are crustaceans with four pairs of legs and one pair of pincers. It's hard to imagine that anyone could have crabs and not know it, but some varieties are small, such as hermit crabs, for instance. Give your swimsuit a close inspection before putting it back on. And watch out for those pincers!

International travel may provide an opportunity to contact a sexually transmitted disease (STD) indigenous only to certain geographic locales. In Australia, for instance, an infestation of pubic *hares* has been wreaking much havoc among the sexually-active outdoor types of that island continent. There is some evidence, still inconclusive, that these pestiferous and really little bunnies are growing in number faster than any other species in the Land of Oz. Caution is advised. *Note:* Although somewhat similar in appearance, the rare pubic *kangaroo* is completely harmless. If you are anticipating overseas outdoor adventure travel, contact the Centers for Disease Control (CDC), International STD Section, in Atlanta, Georgia, for specific warnings and recommended inoculations prior to leaving this country. The CDC maintains a 24-hour phone service: 1 (HOT) SEX-LINE. This same line will also provide you with treatment recommendations if you think you've already contracted some sort of STD. Speak freely. The CDC people are very professional, although some callers report what sounds like good-natured snickering in the background.

You may hear a sexually active female remark about contact with an unusual life form: "That guy last night was a real worm . . . or snake . . . or slug!" Sexually active males are more often overhead talking about something fuzzier: "Man, was she a dog!" It is probably safe to assume that the critters being referred to are sexually transmitted, and, once again, caution is advised.

Of all the STDs, the most common and the fastest spreading is the human papilloma virus (HPV). The interesting name of this virus came from the place where it was first identified, which was Human, Spain. (*Note:* The "H" is silent.) HPV is also known as genital warts, venereal warts, and condyloma. There are at least 60 types of HPV, some causing warts on "private parts" and some causing warts on other parts of the body. The warts can be whitish, brownish, pinkish, or flesh-colorish. They can be as large as a dime or so small they only show up under magnification. They can hurt and itch, but they usually produce no symptoms, which is another one of the reasons why universal precautions don't always work. The virus is highly contagious and can be spread through any kind of genital contact, not just intercourse. All you have to do is rub up against one of the warts. If a female is involved in the relationship, HPV transmission can be prevented with the use of aspirin. One aspirin is placed between the knees of the female, and held there very tightly until the urge to have sex passes. This also works for prevention of pregnancy.

Safety from Parenthood

With due regard for the words of Ed Bluestone—"If God wanted sex to be fun, he wouldn't have invented children as punishment"—there are several ways to prevent pregnancy while still having sex in the outdoors. Most of these methods work just as well indoors and are beyond the scope of this book. But remember, guys, a vasectomy means never having to say you're sorry! And it should probably be noted here, just in passing, that camouflage condoms offer absolutely no more protection outdoors than indoors, even though they are, of course, less noticeable should you accidentally leave one lying around outside the tent. The purpose of cami-condoms is to provide secrecy: No one can see you coming! (*Note:* Cami-condoms are available in Deep Forest, Desert Storm, Boulder, and Duff.)

One method of birth control not suitable for the urban environment, but sometimes successful outdoors, is the cryogenic method. Cryogenics has nothing to do with weeping, but is, instead, the science of cold and cold's effect on things. For the cryogenic method to work it has to be very cold outside. Just before the critical moment, all the insulation must be thrown off and the sperm freezes to death on the way out of the male partner. Timing is very important, and the cryogenic method of birth control has been known to fail, especially with hot-blooded lovers.

Another outdoor method of birth control involves the use of herbal remedies for pregnancy. To work, these herbs must be eaten by the female relatively soon after intercourse. The most popular remedy comes from the seeds of a plant called *Queen Anne's Lace*. Anne, you may remember, was a famous queen who had trouble getting pregnant. Care must be taken to positively identify the plant. Plants, you may also remember, like to mischievously disguise themselves as other plants (see Chapter 7: Environmental Exposure). Queen Anne's Lace is a member of the carrot family and, as such, looks much like the deadly poison *hemlock*, another member of the carrot family. An average adult female must consume approximately 2 million seeds of Queen Anne's Lace per day to insure contraception. Two million seeds weigh about 50 pounds. It is strongly advised to gather the seeds prior to intercourse. The seeds taste terrible, but may be mixed with granola.

Wild yams may also be eaten to prevent pregnancy. In fact, there is a substance in wild yams that is found in many brands of birth control pills. Yams taste much better than the seeds, especially with a little butter and sugar and a bottle of a slightly dry, red dinner wine. Since they require cooking to be palatable, and cooking takes time, use of wild yams should be planned well ahead of time.

Excuse to Avoid: "Not now, William . . . the yams are still boiling!" (*Note:* If you dare follow the advice in the preceding paragraph, go ahead and paint that spare bedroom pink or blue.)

Less Serious Safety Concerns

Many of you know, or at least have heard of, people who think sex is "dirty." Some of those people think sex is dirty because of religious or moral beliefs. Those people are incorrect. The truth is a lot of people just don't keep their sexual stuff as clean from dirt (and germs) as they should. People who think sex is dirty for that reason are often correct.

Urinary Tract Infection

For about 20 percent of all women in the United States, and as many as 5 percent of men, urinary tract infections (UTIs) are akin to a curse. It is more common in women because the urethra, the tube from the bladder to the outdoors, is much shorter in women than in men (or, at least, in many men). A lot of people who have UTIs find it difficult to discuss their problem, since having sex is the most common cause. Bacteria that results in UTIs already lives on and in a person's body, and "going all the way" may move those germs all the way into the urethra. *Note:* UTIs have been associated with whirlpools, swimming pools, and carpools during long commutes, none of which are relevant to the outdoors. Typical signs of UTI include an increased need to urinate, a burning sensation during urination, and low abdominal pain. If you think you have a UTI, you should check out of the North Face "Hilton" and check in with your favorite doctor for some antibiotics. The best ways to prevent UTI are to (1) stay as clean as possible and (2) pee often, especially after having sex. Frequent urination, which is a good idea for everyone, can be encouraged by drinking lots of wine . . . and beer, too.

Testicular Torsion

Testicular Torsion (or "nut" if you were, like me, raised in Georgia) is a twisting of the testicles within the scrotum (or "nut sack," again, if you were raised in Georgia). Activities that cause testicular torsion can be dramatic, such as throwing your partner over your shoulder (as a part of sex and not after sex), or as simple as rolling over in a sleeping bag. The blood supply gets squeezed and the testicles may die if the cut-off of circulation is complete. That's real bad. The pain of a tangled nut is sudden, and intense. The sense of horror to the victim is unimaginable (unless you can imagine, well, never mind).

In Great Britain testicular torsion is known as "getting a knot in your knickers," knickers being a sort of outdoor pant worn by many English gentlemen. The Scots refer to this same condition as "getting a knot in your wee kilty."

You can make it all better by rotating the displaced nut back into its correct position. Since most most testicles rotate inward, a gentle lifting and rotation outward may give immediate and blessed relief. If that didn't work, and someone has passed out, perhaps you've twisted the testicle in the wrong direction. What you should now do is rotate the testicle two turns in the opposite direction. Don't lose count! The affected party may wish to make the adjustment himself, an understandable wish, but men who've had their nuts realigned by a sympathetic, warm-handed partner have been known to bond to that partner in a lasting, forever-grateful fashion.

Vaginitis

Vaginitis is pretty much limited to women—and those women have probably been less than completely hygienic in the outdoors. Unlike a UTI, vaginitis tends to burn and itch all the time. A discharge with an unpleasant odor may be released by the vagina. Over-the-counter medications for the treatment of vaginitis are available and may be purchased ahead of time and carried in an outdoor first aid kit. Treatment also includes (1) staying as clean as possible, and (2) staying naked as much as possible. *Opening Line to Remember:* "If you want to slip out of those clothes and prevent vaginitis, Wilma, I won't mind!"

Prevention of Less Serious Concerns

Since so much safety depends on cleanliness, a few words concerning camp hygiene are in order. Camp hygiene, in this case, refers to regular cleaning of your own nether regions—or the cleaning of another person's nether regions—while camping. This can be accomplished by spending a few moments each day squatting with a bucket or pot of water and a little soap. It should be obvious, but here it is anyway: Washing another person's groin or having another person wash your groin is not a form of birth control. (*Note:* During winter or high-altitude expeditions, snow can be substituted for soap and water. In this case, grime simply freezes and falls off. Care must be taken, however, to prevent other things from freezing and falling off.) In addition, sexual devices should be thoroughly washed and allowed to air dry between uses.

SAFE OUTDOOR SEX COMPARISON CHART

Your best bet for avoiding STDs, pregnancy, and general uncleanness while having sex in the outdoors is to know your partner before you "know" your partner. You can position the odds in your favor by learning whether your potential partner falls into a low-risk or high-risk group.

LOW-RISK GROUPS	HIGH-RISK GROUPS
Backpackers	Backpackers from California with Sierra Club patches on their packs
Mountain biker	Harley Davidson bikers

LOW-RISK GROUPS	HIGH-RISK GROUPS
Canoeists	Canoeists with "Canoeists Do It With Paddles" bumper stickers
Mountain climbers	Rock climbers, especially those wearing tiger-striped Lycra
Car campers	Car campers near Grateful Dead concerts
SCUBA divers	Nude SCUBA divers and oil rig divers
Cowboys	Cowboys from the Bronx
Amateur photographers	Professional photographers
NOLS students	NOLS instructors
Outward Bound instructors	Outward Bound students
U.S.G.S. surveyors	Pipeline surveyors
Remote foreign villagers	Remote foreign villagers who live near U.S. military bases
Church group members	Southern Baptist and Catholic Women's Church group members
Ornithologists	Archeologists
Environmentalists	Environmental lobbyists from Washington, D.C.
Sheep herders	Sheep
National Park Rangers	National Park Outfitters
Large vegetable hunters	Big game hunters
Ginseng gatherers	Mushroom gatherers
Orchid growers	Marijuana growers
Scouts	Scoutmasters
Dogsledders	Snowmobilers
Cross-country skiers	Downhill skiers, especially members of the National Ski Patrol
Loggers	Loggers in bars on Friday night
Prospectors traveling alone	Prospectors traveling with a burro
Writers	Editors

Guidelines for Sex
in the Outdoors

"If it's worth doing, it's worth doing right."

—Anonymous

Creating the Mood

Ambiance is underrated. Do what you can to create a setting conducive to
sex in the outdoors, a mood of quiet comfort and easy intimacy delicately
balanced with profound anticipation. Start the campfire early, so it has a
chance to burn down to a soft, crackling glow. Use resinous woods for the
fire, for example, pine and fir. Alder and cottonwood smell bad. (*Note:* If you
have a not-so-fit body, place the fire far away from the tent. You don't want
too much light.) Place the wine in a creek or lake to chill. (*Note:* In the
absence of creeks and lakes, you can wrap the wine in a wet T-shirt. Evapo-
ration will chill it admirably.) Consider decanting the wine into a water bottle before serving. Decanting allows the wine to breathe, and allows you to

hide the fact that you bought a half-gallon of Red Goofy that was on sale for $3.98. (*Note:* If you bought good wine, skip decanting, and leave the price tag visible.) Open the can of smoked oysters in time to wash off the stinky juice that invariably spills all over your hands. Make sure your last dump was well away from the tent, and downwind, and wash up profusely afterwards.

Preparing the Boudoir

Boudoir is technically French for a "woman's private room," but calling the tent that helps set the mood. *Opening Line to Remember:* "Shall we retire to the boudoir, my dear?" Unroll the sleeping pads and lay on them, checking for lumps. Remove the lumps. Unstuff the sleeping bags early, so they have time to fluff up. Shake out the pine needles from the last trip. If you brought a book of poetry, place it—and a flashlight—near at hand. (Robert Service, perhaps, for the traditionalist, or Billy Collins for the trendy. Dirty limericks for the ultra-trendy.) Make sure there's a fresh candle in the candle lantern. Place a fresh roll of toilet paper near the tent door.

What He Wants Her to Know

It ain't the same for me as it is for you, but I sure wish it was! It doesn't take much to turn me on . . . almost anything will do it . . . like a glimpse of your fresh-washed underwear drying on a bush. That doesn't mean I don't respect you, or think of you, especially parts of you, as less than a person. Well, maybe it does a little bit . . . but not much! I can feel that way about your body parts and still care about you deeply. It's just that thinking about those things gets the old ball rolling. Maybe you find this hard to understand.

Part of the problem is this: You can just lie there and do it, if you have to, without much interest, but I have to have some stimulus to get the "old feller" up for the occasion. If I don't get turned on, nothing happens. I can't be "taken" or "used" like you can . . . at least not in the same way. Most of what I physically feel is in my private parts. Maybe that's why I grab for one of your private parts right away. You say you need time to get "in the mood," but grabbing parts is how I get in the mood. Maybe you could teach me how to feel with other parts.

You think I think of you as a sex object. That's true sometimes, but what I'd really like is for you to think of me, now and then, as a sex object. How about putting some of that "women's intuition" into intuiting that I'd like for you, every once in a while, to be the aggressor, to start grabbing before I do. Wouldn't that be fun? It would be for me, anyway. Hey, we're way out here in the woods . . . who's gonna know?

I think the best lover would be one who stays "all woman" but jumps in about half the time like a man would. The best lover doesn't make ugly faces when I undress, doesn't attract moose with during-sex noises, doesn't fall asleep during sex, has multiple orgasms, and is well trained in wilderness medicine.

What She Wants Him to Know

Just because it takes me longer to get going doesn't mean I don't care. If you're willing to take time, instead of wham-bam-thank-you-ma'am, then I know that you care, too. I get excited sometimes by being casually touched and by seeing male parts, but it seems like it takes me longer for things to build up. It appears to me as if you can get completely satisfied in a few minutes, but I can't do that. Sometimes I'm excited but you're too blind to see it, and I don't have the visible display you have to announce it. I get interested in having sex by being involved with your personality, by the unpredictable (and gentle) things you do to me, by the mood that is created when we're together.

There are a lot of times when I don't do things to you because I'm afraid of your reaction. What would really help me is if you told me things you'd like for me to do. I don't think women's intuition is as powerful as you think it is. It seems like you expect me to read your mind. I don't mind being the aggressor sometimes, but I like being aggressed, too.

But don't be cruel! Sometimes sex in the outdoors can be pretty wild, but it should never be mean or unkind. I *am* a person and I *am* an equal. Sometimes I get really frustrated by you, by your rush and your lack of gentleness, but I think I very seldom show it.

I think the best lover is one who is sensitive to the individual woman I am. The best lover doesn't have an orgasm while undressing, always removes his boots first, is comfortable in at least five different positions, doesn't get distracted by nearby bellowing moose, doesn't keep asking "How's it going?," has multiple orgasms, and gives long back rubs *after* sex.

Après-Sex

Consider what you say immediately after sex. It can have a very negative or positive effect on the next time.

Some bad choices of après-sex statements include but are not limited to: (1) Ha-ha! Do you call that an orgasm? (2) Uh-oh, the condom ripped! (3) Thanks a bunch! I was saving that banana for breakfast. (4) I didn't realize you had put on so much weight. (5) My last sexual partner was much better. (6) What's that awful smell? (7) Is that it? (8) I'm ready for some shuteye. How 'bout you? (9) Hand me the first-aid kit! (10) Maybe you were just nervous. (11) Hey, get it yourself! (12) I could get it up and/or wet again, but I choose not to. (13) Where's my glass eye? (14) Thank you very much.

Some good choices of après-sex statements include but are not limited to: (1) It was never like that before! (2) I didn't know it could last that long. (3) You smell wonderful. (4) You taste wonderful. (5) How do you hold your breath so long? (6) Is your tongue licensed as a deadly weapon? (7) How did you get so flexible? (8) I'm glad you forgot your sleeping bag. (9) Do you want to try that indoors sometime? (10) Let's hold hands and watch the moon rise. (11) I'm not the least bit sleepy. (12) Are you ready to go again? (13) Thank you very much.

Some après-sex statements that could go either way include but are not limited to: (1) Did you have the big O? (2) Where's the toilet paper? (3) Your T-shirt's on upside down. (4) Are you hungry? (5) Are these your socks? (6) I didn't know they made inflatable condoms. (7) When did you start shaving your pubic hair? (8) Would you like to meet my mom and dad? (9) Do you always scream like that? (10) You're better than I heard you were. (11) You're sure able to do a lot with so little. (12) Will you untie me now? (13) Thank you very much.

The Most Important Guideline

Have fun!

12

Testimonials:
We Did It Our Way

"Experience is a cruel and heartless teacher."

Yes, sex in the outdoors does happen, as these testimonials will further illustrate. Whether they turn you on or turn you off, entertain you or bore you, there is almost always something to be learned from the experiences of others.

Rising to the Occasion

"J and I reached the summit of Mexico's 5,452 meter (18,882 feet) Popocatépetl on New Year's Day. Popo, a smoking volcano, is named for a famous Aztec hero who still 'carries the torch' for his dead love, Iztaccihuatl, whose name is stuck on another nearby volcano. Down below, at Tlamacas Lodge, hundreds of people were celebrating. We had climbed a route called Las Cruces and, looking back, we could see lots of climbers coming up the same route. But we had started yes-

Testimonials: We Did It Our Way **95**

terday, camped just below snow line, and topped out early. We were the only ones on the summit that morning. J and I had been going out for a couple of months, back in Montana, and it wasn't too hard to talk her into a 'quickie,' to honor the spirit of Popo, and to celebrate this special occasion. There's a summit hut on Popocatépetl, but we discarded that idea after a brief glimpse of its broken-down interior. We used the hut as a windbreak and did what we call 'sitting-sex'—I sat on my pack, and she, well, anyway, it totally took my breath away in a very literal way. I'm glad we did it. It makes fond memories and a good story. But my final analysis of sex at 18,000 feet is that it's more a matter of survival than fun."

—*BS, Missoula, Montana*

A Rustling in the Leaves

"Here in Georgia the leaves on the oak trees turn brown and fall to carpet the forest floor every autumn. It sure is pretty, and it smells kinda good when you pile 'em up and roll around in the pile. My boyfriend and me like to roll around in piles of leaves, and sometimes that leads to other things. My family lives on the edge of the woods, and we don't have to walk very far to find enough leaves to rake into a big pile. We were doing 'other things' one Saturday afternoon when I heard Pa call my name. He sounded real close. I peeked up and saw he wasn't far away, but he was looking the other way. So we quietly packed a lot of leaves over us, and we lay real still. Before long Pa went back to the house. We got dressed and walked back real casual, like nothing had happened. P.S. If y'all try this, we recommend you bring a blanket because the leaves are scratchy."

—*Bobby Jean, Albany, Georgia*

Beach Blanket Bango

"Sand is always a challenge, dudes. The challenge is to keep the sand out of your eyes, nose, and other moist places where it causes itching and discomfort. After years of excellent experiences, I'd like to offer two pieces of advice. One, wait, if you can, for low tide, and use the inter-tidal zone where the sand is damp and compacted.

Timing is important so you don't get washed out to sea. Two, use a very large blanket, dudes. Both of these pieces of advice are virtually useless if the wind is blowing. If the wind is blowing, use the lifeguard hut."

—*Hunk Harrison, lifeguard, Palm Beach, California*

Stiff Ride

"My friends, they call me Madman because I'll try anything once, just for the hell of it, especially on my mountain bike. Not long ago some of the guys bet me I couldn't actually have sex with my girl while actually riding my bike. Well, my girl, you could call her Madwoman because she's almost as crazy as me, she said OK. We practiced some positions, sitting on a stool in the kitchen, and picked one with me on the bike seat and her on me. There's an old dirt road through the woods not far from town, and that's where we did it. The road was bumpy and that helped. It wasn't really that good—and don't tell anybody that—but I won the bet. I want to tell you this, though, if you decide to try it, you should keep your eyes on the road."

—*Room 151, Franklin Memorial Hospital, Philadelphia, Pennsylvania*

Bare Attack (edited for publication)

"There was just the two of us hiking in grizzly country. After dinner we had turned off the stove and we were talking quietly in the dark when the urge struck. We were going at it pretty hard, near the fire (which had died down), on a foamlite pad, with her on top, when suddenly she screamed. Screaming wasn't something she normally did, so I opened my eyes. I was just in time to witness a huge grizzly bear snatching her off me and dragging her into the woods. I have heard the smell of sex can attract a bear. Anyway, I never saw her again. I was embarrassed to tell the truth before now. Everybody thinks she just wandered off alone and never showed up again."

—*Anonymous Person, Anonymous Town, Anonymous State*

On the Rocks: Version One

"TJ and I were visiting the Garden of the Gods near Colorado Springs when we decided to scramble up a tall stack of boulders not far from the Visitor Center. There was one place where I had to give her a boost up a tricky spot. TJ is shorter than I am, and she couldn't reach the next ledge, but she insisted we keep going. From the top we could look down and see climbers with ropes and harnesses working their way up another steeper side. It was a warm summer day, and TJ thought we could work in a little sex before the other climbers reached the top. I was nervous, but that part worked fine! But we heard the noise of the climbers and realized they were almost there while we were still naked. So we hurried, with our clothes in our arms, down the side we had come up. At the tricky spot we dropped our clothes and I jumped down. But TJ, still being shorter, was afraid to make the jump. She had to lie down and slowly slide over the edge, scraping off some skin, and letting her legs down until I could reach them. This was accompanied by some very appreciative calls from the climbers. TJ loves to tell this story at parties."

—*Bob, Pitkin, Colorado*

On the Rocks: Version Two

"Bob and I stopped to see the Garden of the Gods, near Colorado Springs, one summer day, and he decided we should try to climb up a very dangerous rock formation near the Visitor Center. Other people were climbing the same rocks, sensibly using ropes to protect themselves. At one point it was so steep I told him we should turn back,

but he insisted we keep climbing. He had to lift me up so I could climb over the really steep part. Once on the top, he practically tore my clothes off, telling me how exciting sex up there would be. I finally gave in when he said if I didn't he would climb down and leave me. When he was almost done, the climbers came up over the edge. We grabbed our clothes and ran for it. But at the really steep place he jumped down and left me. If I had not screamed, I am sure he would have deserted me. Finally, he came back up and helped me down. But I got some very bad abrasions on sensitive areas. The climbers seemed to think it was all great fun. I hate it when Bob tells this story at parties."

—*TJ, Pitkin, Colorado*

Wet Dreams

"A couple of years ago some totally cool friends I had just met at school, and me, decided to run the San Juan River, the stretch from Mexican Hat on down toward Lake Powell. It was Spring Break. As the sun got hotter and hotter, we kept taking off clothes until all of us were naked and really having a totally cool time. The girl sitting next to me, I forget her name, kept rubbing up against me, and we kept getting hotter and hotter, and the beer was flowing almost as fast as the river (and some other stuff), until, I don't remember when it started, she was sitting on my lap, and we were doing the wild thing. It was totally cool, especially in the rapids. The only downer was this jerk sitting on the side of the river by a canoe who kept staring at us through binoculars."

—*X, Logan, Utah*

Howdah Do It on an Elephant

"Please, I would not say this thing, but my good friend, Mr. Buck, has asked me to say something. So let me tell you that I am a guide in India who takes the Americans on rides on the elephant's back in very nice howdahs, I think, with cushions. There are some times when I take others who are my good friends on rides on the elephant's back when there are not the tourists to take. Sometimes we do more than only ride and let me tell you, please, that the elephant's back sways and bumps most delightfully. It is not necessary to move, because, you see, the elephant moves for both of us. Once, I must tell you, this can be most embarrassing for the elephant when you do not guide him, for then he walks where he wishes, even into the streets of the city. Mr. Buck has also asked me to say that he has not tried this and he is my good friend also. Thank you."

—*No name, please, Mumbai, India*

Howls in the Desert

"We, George and I (maybe you should leave George's name off of this), had been hiking with a guided group in the desert country of Arizona for almost two weeks when we thought it was time to slip away, one night, to reestablish our sexual relationship. The moon was bright and it was a fairly warm night, and we were squirming around partly on the sleeping bags and partly off. Suddenly, George started howling like something straight out of hell. I jumped up and saw a scorpion rushing off. It had stung him right on the bum. He howled for about 10 minutes before he finally calmed down. I know it must have hurt, but I couldn't stop laughing. The really funny part was that several members of the group commented the next day on how active the coyotes had been that night. George recovered, but our relationship didn't."

—Funny Girl, Prescott, Arizona

Rolling on the Sea

 "As a physician with a private practice, I have had to deal with all kinds of pathologies (sickness). This is one of my least favorite stories, but perhaps some of your readers may benefit from it. Before my wife and I bought our sailboat, we rented a small one out of Honolulu, and, on the first night, anchored in a semi-protected cove south of the city. Since it was our first night on board, we thought we should celebrate by having intercourse (sex) on the deck. The swells were rolling us gently but consistently, back and forth, up and down, back and forth. At first the rising and falling of the sea seemed to increase the pleasure of intercourse, but, all of a sudden, I felt an involuntary bolus of emesis (puke) rising. This required an immediate withdrawal, but, unable to make the railing, I spewed all over the deck. I would, therefore, strongly recommend an acclimatization period—or, at least, a strong anti-vertigo (motion sickness) drug—before attempting sex at sea."

—MD, New York, New York

A Branching of Limbs

"G'day, mate. Here in the Land of Oz, we've got the most dangerous creatures in the whole world. The most poisonous snakes live here, and the most poisonous spiders, not to mention a bloody hell of a tangle of giant lizards and meddlesome 'roos. And that's just on land. The bloody sea is filled with giant, man-eating sharks, and poisonous jellyfish, and bloody poisonous octopussies. What's a mate to do for a bit of outdoor mating? Some of us, yeah, we've gone to the trees. Down Under we've got kilometer after bloody kilometer of eucalyptus trees.

Me and a mate were up a giant eucalyp just the other day when the mate wanted to mate. It takes a bit of balancing, it does, but when you get the hang of it, you'll be hard on to top it. It's a lovely boppy, especially when the tree sways in the wind.

—Emil, Perth, Western Australia

Sex in the Outdoors

second edition

APPENDIXES

Appendix I:
Other Ways to Say "Have Sex"

"A rose, by any other name, would smell as sweet."

—W. SHAKESPEARE.

SCIENTIFIC WAYS:

1. Intercourse

2. Copulation

3. Coitus

4. Procreation

5. Fornication

SOCIALLY-ACCEPTABLE WAYS:

1. Messing around

2. Fooling around

3. Playing around

4. Going to bed

5. Sleeping together

6. Merging

7. Uniting

8. Going all the way

9. Making love

MARGINALLY-ACCEPTABLE WAYS:

1. Doing it

2. Doing the serious

3. Doing the act

4. Doing the deed

5. Poking

6. Laying

7. Getting laid

Unacceptable Ways:

1. Screwing
2. Fornication under carnal knowledge
3. Humping
4. Getting a piece of ass
5. Going down
6. Getting some
7. Balling
8. Nailing
9. Playing circus

Archaic Ways:

1. Making babies
2. Knowing someone (in the Biblical sense)

Cute Ways:

1. Bumping uglies
2. Bumping fuzzies
3. Hiding the salami
4. The old in-and-out
5. Bopping
6. Doing the horizontal bop
7. The wild thing
8. Doing the laundry (small loads)
9. Making the beast with two backs

Sports Ways:

1. Scoring
2. Getting to fourth base
3. Hitting a homerun
4. Touchdown
5. Slamdunk

MILITARY WAYS:

1. Sinking the torpedo (Navy)
2. Dropping the bomb (Air Force)
3. Firing one in (Army)
4. Beach Blanket Bingo (Marines)
5. Interdiction (Coast Guard)

Appendix 2:
Views of Outdoor Sex by World Religions

"Think with the whole body."

—TAISEN DESHIMARU

TAOISM: Sex in the outdoors happens.

CONFUCIANISM: Confucius say, "Sex in the outdoors happens."

BUDDHISM: If sex in the outdoors happens, it isn't really sex.

ZEN BUDDHISM: What is the sound of sex in the outdoors happening?

HINDUISM: This sexual experience has happened before.

ISLAM: If sex in the outdoors happens, it is the Will of Allah.

SOUTHERN BAPTISM: Sex in the outdoors happens, but not on Sunday.

METHODISM: If sex in the outdoors happens, feel guilty.

CATHOLICISM: If sex in the outdoors happens, feel guilty, and ask for forgiveness.

MORMONISM *(for men)*: Sex in the outdoors happens, with multiple partners.

MORMONISM *(for women)*: Sex in the outdoors happens, but not often enough.

JUDAISM: Why doesn't sex in the outdoors ever happen to us?

SHINTOISM: Sex happens everywhere, but it's best outdoors!

Appendix 3: Rules for Outdoor Sex

"Women would rather be right than reasonable."

—OGDEN NASH

Decided upon via consensus by the Women of America's League for the Propagation of Sex in the Outdoors (WALPSO) after very little deliberation, this codification represents the only written order of conduct for outdoor sex. Almost all the cultures of the world, however, have oral traditions, passed down from generation to generation, that say pretty much the same thing.

1. Women always make The Rules for sex in the outdoors.

2. Men can never ever know all The Rules.

3. The Rules are always subject to change at any time without prior notification.

4. If a Woman thinks a Man knows all The Rules, she must immediately change some or all of The Rules.

5. Women are never wrong.

6. If it seems like the Woman is wrong, it is due to a misunderstanding that was a direct result of something the Man did or said that was wrong.

7. The Man should apologize immediately for causing the misunderstanding.

8. The Woman, at any time, may change her mind about having sex in the outdoors.

9. The Man may never change his mind without the expressed written consent of the Woman.

10. The Woman has every right to be angry, upset, and frustrated at any time by any sexual experience in the outdoors.

11. The Man must remain calm at all times unless the Woman wants him to be angry, upset, and frustrated.

12. The Woman must not, under any circumstances, let the Man know whether or not she wants him to be angry, upset, and/or frustrated.

13. The Man is expected to read the Woman's mind.

14. The Woman is ready for sex in the outdoors when she is ready.

15. The Man must be ready at all times.

16. If the Woman has Pre-Menstrual Syndrome (PMS), all The Rules are null and void.

17. Any Man who doesn't abide by The Rules can't take the heat, lacks backbone, and is a wimp.

Sex in the Outdoors

Appendix 4: The Chemistry of Outdoor Sex

"Sex is a romantic designation for a most ordinary biological—or, shall we say, chemical?—process. A lot of nonsense is talked and written about."

almost what Greta Garbo said in *Ninotchka*

Thinking about sex, preparing for sex, having sex, recovering from sex—they all produce a lot of stress. And well they should, since the chemical pathways for both, inside the human body, are the same. All of that sweat, panting, and flushing of the skin (the things you love!) are caused by chemicals that your body produces, chemicals that are first-cousins to amphetamines (uppers): dopamine, norepinephrine, and phenylethylamine. The reaction of those chemicals in your body—the euphoria—unfortunately, doesn't last very long. That's why people so often feel a letdown after having sex.

There's another chemical involved inside the bodies of people who start feeling really attached to each other. Long-lasting relationships are built on increased production of endorphins, the human body's natural painkiller, which causes soothing emotions like peace, security, and tranquility. The internal production of those chemicals, sadly, will start to peter out over time, too.

One more chemical you should know about is oxytocin, the "cuddle chemical." Oxytocin, manufactured by human brains, makes mothers want to cuddle their babies, and it makes men and women want to cuddle up. It also makes orgasms better. Oxytocin production increases three to five times as one nears climax.

Why do you need to know this? Because *Dr. Rose's Outdoor Sex Pills* contain more than twice the Recommended Daily Allowance (RDA) of phenylethylamine and endorphins and oxytocin! Yes, *Dr. Rose's Outdoor Sex Pills* can rekindle the old spark and give you the lift you need to keep going. *Dr. Rose's Outdoor Sex Pills* come in fast-release, easy-to-swallow capsules for that power punch you desire. And they dissolve quickly in wine, without leaving a traceable residue or after-taste. *Dr. Rose's Outdoor Sex Pills* are guaranteed to work, or your money happily refunded. Use the order form enclosed with this book to order today! Ask for *Dr. Rose's Outdoor Sex Pills!*

Warnings! Use only as directed. This product has never been tested indoors.

Note: The preceding is a paid advertisement.

Appendix 5: Suggested Reading

"Reading rots the mind."

—EDWARD ABBEY

Anonymous. *Debbie Does Denali*. Talkeetna, AK: Mount and Press, 1983. (*Note:* This is part of an exciting new series that includes *Bob Bops the Boundary Waters* and *Edna Eats the Everglades*.)

Bechtel, Stefan. *The Practical Encyclopedia of Sex and Health: From Aphrodisiacs and Hormones to Potency, Stress, Vasectomy and Yeast Infection*. Emmaus, PA: Rodale, Inc., 1993.

Butts, Seymour. Nudist Colonies: *Behind the Scenes*. Wacko, TX: Moon Publishers, 2001.

Concolor, Felis. *My Sex Life with a Mountain Man*. Unpublished manuscript, 1839.

Discomfort, Alex, MS (Master of Sex). *The Pain of Outdoor Sex: Getting the Point of Pine Needles*. Sincinnati, OH: Ohmygosh Press, 2000.

Editors (The) of *Men's Health*. *Sexercise for Men*. Emmaus, PA: Rodale, Inc., 1996.

Katz, Jeremy, et al. *Report 2004: A Man's Guide to Women*. Emmaus, PA: Rodale, Inc., 2004.

Katz, Bunny, et al. *Report 2004: A Woman's Guide to Men*. Paradise, NV: Bodacious, Inc., 2004.

Miller, D. *Anatomy of Human Genitalia: A Guide in Words and Lurid Pictures*. Wuaneta, NE: Nasty Publishing Company, 2002.

Pain and Suffering. "The elasticity of the vagina versus the elasticity of the anus compared via the insertion of increasingly larger objects into volunteers who first swore on a stack of Bibles not to reveal their identities." *The Journal of Sex in the Outdoors,* Vol. 1, Number 1, Nov. 2003.

Secret, Victoria. *Crotchless Long Undies, and Other Outdoor Sex-Wear: A Buyer's Guide.* Temptation, AZ: Wash and Wear Press, 2002.

Tilton, Buck. *Deep Throat* An interview recorded by the author on November 5, 1968, and subsequently locked in a vault in Lander, WY.

Winthrope, M. *Sex Slave: How to Find One, How to Be One.* Watertown, MA: Ivory Tower Publishing Company, Inc., 1991.

Glossary of Sex-Related Terms

From *Merriam-Websters Collegiate Dictionary*—glossary: a collection of textual glosses or of specialized terms with their meanings. *also see* glossa[from the Greek]: a tongue or lingual structure...[especially useful in the outdoors].

AIDS,

a mighty unwelcome visitor, see Chapter 10

Anal intercourse,

the road less traveled

Aphrodisiac,

something that makes him/her look a lot better, see Chapter 8

Bestiality,

a practice requiring breadcrumbs, hay, or raw meat, see Chapter 8

Boob,

anyone not interested in this book

Boudoir,

wherever you land, see Chapter 11

Breast,

not the white meat of a chicken

Buns,

not something that goes well with the white meat of a chicken

Butt,

see Buns

Canadian Bureau of Outdoor Sex Standards (CBOSS),

an office in Canada

Centers for Disease Control (CDC),

an office in Atlanta

Clitoris,

what she wants her partner to find

Condom,

something carried in your wallet or your tampon case, see Chapter 10

Copulation,

see *Merriam-Webster*'s Dictionary

Crouching,

use your imagination

Debbie Does Denali,

see X-rated

Denali Does Debbie,

see XXX-rated

Erotic pictures,

a vision generally relegated to your mind

Fondling,

a welcome and gentle squeezing

Genito-urinary,

look in your shorts

Horny,

look in the mirror

Hydration,

the result of drinking something

"It,"

what this book is all about

Ligottage,

a French term for a knotty situation

Masturbation,

for when the advice in Chapter 4 fails

Mating,

a good thing for people and socks

Ménage à trois,

a real good thing for people, bad for socks

Nudity,

the outfit you come in

Nut sack,

the ball carrier

Oral sex,

a kind of hygiene

Orgasm,

the reward for a job well done

Outdoor Bondage Safety Code,

something to be followed without fail

Peak Experience,

hey, isn't "it" always supposed to be that way, see Chapter 7

Peek Experience,

a poor relative of a Peak Experience, see Chapter 8

Pecker,

not another name for a chicken

Penis,

what he wants his partner to find

Phallic shock,

his first time, see Chapter 7

Poke,

not a kind of salad

Pornographic,

referring to something you wish he or she was more of

Reproduction,

a result of unsafe sex

Scrotum,

see nut sack

Sex,

the reason for this book

Shit,

something always done 200 feet away from any sexual activity

Soixante-neuf,

a French term for a shared meal

Sport-bra,

outdoor breast-hiding device

Teats (Tits),

archaic, see Boob

Testicular torsion,

something way down on the list of preferred personal experiences

Vagina,

anagram of navigate without the "t" or "e"

Vasectomy,

a term men use when they can't find a condom

Virginity,

not the capitol of Nevada

Voyeurism,

when a peek is all you get, see Chapter 8

"Wild Kingdom,"

the unwashed groin

"Wild Thing,"

see "sex;" not to be confused with "Wild Kingdom"

X-rated,

may apply to hot sauce or hiking shorts, see Debbie Does Denali

XXX-rated,

may apply to hot sauce or hiking shorts, see Denali Does Debbie